Magic on Mira Road
Stories from the Bhaktivedanta Hospital

Radha Bhakti Dasi

All profits from the sale of this book are donated to the
Bhaktivedanta Hospital, Mira Road, Mumbai, India

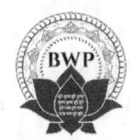

Bookwrights Press
Charlottesville, VA

Copyright © 2026 Radha Bhakti Dasi (Rashi Singh)
All Rights Reserved
No part of this publication can be reproduced in any form without prior permission of the author and publisher.

Published by

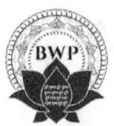

Bookwrights Press
Charlottesville, VA USA
bookwrightspress. com
publisher@bookwrightspress.com

All profits from the sale of this book are donated to the
Bhaktivedanta Hospital
Mira Road, Mumbai, India

Distributed in India by Tulsi Books
tulsibooks.com

Photos courtesy of the Bhaktivedanta Hospital and the author
Text and cover design by Mayapriya devi dasi

ISBN: 978-1-880404-62-1
Available also as an ebook

Contents

Foreword	v
Introduction	1
Part One: Touching Ground	
A journal entry by the author upon arriving at the Bhaktivedanta Hospital	21
Part Two: Breaking Ground	
Interviews with two Founding Doctors and two Trustees	37
Part Three: On the Ground	
Author's personal journal entries and interviews with the staff and patients of the Bhaktivedanta Hospital	75
Epilogue	221
Acknowledgments	245

❧ ❧ ❧ ❧
Foreword

The Bhaktivedanta Hospital is a project that is very dear to me. I have been treated there a number of times, and have observed a certain magic that is hard to describe. Put simply—it is a place for all to heal physically, emotionally, and spiritually. It is a place that not only provides healthcare, but also inspires people to change their paradigms, to allow the spiritual to supersede the material.

That is why I wanted a writer to interview staff and patients, and to document their stories into a book, which you now have before you: *Magic on Mira Road—Stories from the Bhaktivedanta Hospital*.

I trust that everyone who reads this book will get a glimpse into the power of care based on universal spiritual principles. My teacher, His Divine Grace A. C. Bhaktivedanta Swami Srila Prabhupada, the founder-*acharya*[1] of the International Society for Krishna Consciousness (ISKCON), always wanted us to use our inclinations in service to God, and to the real self, the soul. In this book, you'll be able to see how the Bhaktivedanta Hospital brings this vision to life, in a deeply inspiring way.

Niranjana Swami
January 2025
Mayapur, India

---

1. *Acharya* is one who teaches by example. Founder-*Acharya* is the foremost exemplar, whose teachings all other teachers follow ongoingly, even after his passing.

✤ ✤ ✤ ✤

Introduction

"Daddy, I can't breathe."

My father heard me say this to him more times than he can remember when I was young. I would hobble into my parents' bedroom, gasping for air. I'd wake up my father, and he would hurriedly grab his car keys and rush me to the hospital, still wearing his pyjamas. I was diagnosed with asthma at the age of five. I remember having frequent asthma attacks, always at night. I remember being in the hospital, a lot. I remember being afraid, calling out for my parents or my older sister. I remember feeling special because whenever I was in the hospital my mother used to bring me my favourite meals. And even now as an adult, with my asthma generally under control, I mostly remember the nurses and doctors who were kind, and those who I remember for making me cry.

I suppose most people are uncomfortable in hospitals, being surrounded by so much sickness and death. For me, even when going to the hospital for a good reason, like the birth of my nephews, I've always felt uneasy around the smells, the sounds, the sadness. The impersonalism.

That was why I had a number of reservations when, in 2013, I was presented with an opportunity to volunteer at the Bhaktivedanta Hospital in Mumbai, India. Specifically, I was asked to travel from Canada to India to collect the stories of patients and staff at the Bhaktivedanta Hospital, and put them into a book. The thought was equal parts exhilarating and terrifying; I've always wanted to write a book, but would I really be okay with being surrounded by sickness, sorrow, and death?

A number of events led me to ultimately accept the opportunity. It all started in September of 2012, when my role at a swanky Toronto-based digital marketing agency was made redundant. I considered it a blessing; I had been feeling burnt out and was in need of some sort of rejuvenation. A change of scenery, to say the least.

I wasn't sure what I would do next, but I knew it would involve travel. One day as I was cleaning out my bookshelf, I came across a flyer for the Sandipani Muni School, which is a school for impoverished children located in Vrindavan, India. I didn't know much about the school, and I had no idea how that flyer landed on my bookshelf, but I was intrigued. I had been to Vrindavan many times before, but only for a few days at a time. It was somewhere I was longing to spend more time.

Vrindavan is a major pilgrimage site for the Hare Krishna community, infused with gorgeous forests, bodies of holy waters, farms, and temples. Every corner has another stunning temple; not always stunning because of its size or grandeur, but often because of its simplicity and character.

In contrast, Vrindavan's Krishna-Balarama Mandir—the sacred temple-complex of the Hare Krishna movement—is big, meticulous in its design, and features a large temple room as well as a restaurant and guesthouse. Still, the atmosphere there, for me, is the most devotional, spiritual, and peaceful. As much as I fancied myself a city girl, I always felt more natural and at home in the village of Vrindavan, and yearned to spend more quality time there. The residents of Vrindavan often lived in the simplest, sometimes dire, circumstances. But I'd never seen happiness in anyone as I did in the villagers of Vrindavan. Thus, the notion of volunteering at the Sandipani Muni School in Vrindavan was more appealing than ever before.

A few weeks later, I sublet my apartment, packed a suitcase, and ventured to Vrindavan to volunteer as a teacher and management consultant at the school. I had booked a two-month trip, but ended up staying for four. Needless to say, it was a life-altering experience—one that created an undeniable urge in me to return to India.

But first, I returned to Toronto in March of 2013, unsure of my next move. I felt that simply going back to work would somehow dishonour my experience; how could my life be so deeply affected, only to come back to a corporate life in downtown Toronto? I loved my life before India—I just didn't know if I was ready to go back to it. I was seriously contemplating returning to India in the fall, but I wasn't sure if it was feasible. To keep all my options open, I also began job searching.

All at once, I received a job offer, a request from the school in Vrindavan to come back, and an opportunity to do some work with the Bhaktivedanta Hospital in Mumbai. To have so many doors open at once was rare for me—I could feel something special was in the air.

The opportunity in Mumbai was fascinating. A monk from the Hare Krishna tradition, Niranjana Swami, had written about the Bhaktivedanta Hospital on his blog. I hadn't heard much about the hospital before. From the blog, I learned that it is a holistic care facility that offers care for its patients' bodies, minds, and souls, based on universal spiritual principles as espoused in the ancient yoga text *Bhagavad-gita As It Is*. According to this blog post, so many transformations of heart have occurred within the hospital walls, due to the exceptional care provided by its entire staff. Niranjana Swami put a call out for a writer to collect the stories of staff and patients, and write them down in a book.

This would be a dream come true for me, but I really didn't think it would be feasible, nor did I think I had the ability. What did I know about writing a book? At the insistence of a couple of good friends, I contacted the Swami and told him I'd be interested in helping as part of a team—perhaps I could edit interviews, or conduct some online. He was kind, encouraging, and gracious. After little consideration, I made up my mind: I was going to do this. I could start in Vrindavan at the school for a spiritually uplifting experience, and then go to Mumbai to work at the hospital. It turned out, no one else had come forward; I would do this on my own. I accepted the job offer on a contract basis and then in the fall of 2013, I booked a one-way ticket to India, and off I went.

The book you hold now is the fruit of over a decade's work of bringing the story of the Bhaktivedanta Hospital to life in these pages, in service to the hospital team, and to you.

As soon as I arrived and understood the greatness of the Bhaktivedanta Hospital, I strongly felt that all my life experiences led me to, and equipped me for, my experience at the hospital in January of 2014 onwards. (After spending six months in India, I'd go back at the end of 2014 for a few months and conduct additional interviews.) Every single heartbreak, triumph, relationship, and experience suddenly made sense, and I realized this was where I was meant to be, and writing this book, regardless of how many hands it will reach, was what I was meant to do as a service. I realized quickly that this project had little to do with me; I was just an incredibly fortunate instrument, meant to share the hospital's beautiful story. Over the course of two visits and a cumulative stay of about two months, I interviewed over a hundred staff members, volunteers, patients, and their family members. I'm deeply grateful to everyone who took the time to meet with me. Sadly, I was only able to include some of their stories in this book.

This Introduction attempts to provide context for the philosophy behind the hospital. The next three sections contain the origin story of the hospital, the stories of staff and patients, as well as some of my personal journal entries from my time at the hospital. Each story is written in the voice of the interviewee. I conclude with an Epilogue, outlining events that have taken place since this book project began.

It's worth noting that all stories have been edited for grammar, clarity, and flow, and some were translated from Hindi. Many names, including those of staff, patients, their families, and various institutions, have been changed to protect privacy. In order to understand the stories of the people featured in this book, some additional context is required. The Bhaktivedanta Hospital was founded by four young Hare Krishna devotees, and the tenets by which the hospital operates are based on Hare Krishna principles.

ᴗ ᴗ ᴗ ᴗ

A Crash Course in the Hare Krishna Tradition

I have been a Hare Krishna my entire life. When I say that to people, they usually respond by saying, "Cool, what's that all about?" Once in a while, I hear a bit of "Get a job!" or "Why don't you have a shaved head and wear orange robes?" or "But you're so normal!" (That one's my favourite.) I'm also sometimes asked if I'm part of a cult. This section, and the rest of this Introduction, will explain the context of the tradition, and is not meant to be an imposition on the reader. This tradition is incredibly rich and deep, so in this section we will include only what we feel will help you understand the nuances and the language of the stories in this book. Moreover, it will illuminate the driving force behind the transformations of heart that take place at the hospital.

In the Hare Krishna, or *bhakti-yoga* tradition, practitioners follow a lineage that goes back thousands of years; it is known as Vaishnavism, and has its origins in India. One of the main premises of the tradition is that we are all created equal. We are not our bodies, but rather we are spirit souls that reside *in* our bodies. The soul is eternal, always happy, and completely knowledgeable about its loving relationship with the Divine. Death is merely the movement of the soul from one type of body to another. We could move into a human body, or into the body of any kind of living entity, and live a particular type of life. Our destination and future life are dependent on our consciousness at the time of death, which is determined by our activities and the consciousness we cultivate throughout our current life.

Whether we are Black, Asian, Hindu, Jewish, Canadian, Egyptian, gay, straight, a lawyer, a doctor, or whatever, we are all spirit souls, and we all have the same goal—to remember and revive our dormant love for God, who has many names. Krishna, Allah, Jehovah, and Yahweh are all names of God. In *bhakti*, we most commonly refer to him as Krishna, meaning "All Attractive." In this life, I am a Canadian female management consultant of Indian descent, but in my next life, I could just as easily be an American male doctor of African descent. In fact, I could even take on an animal's body. Therefore, according to *bhakti*, these types of designations (sex, nationality, occupation, etc.), are temporary. Because they belong to the body, these designations can change after death (and in many cases, even during life!), and are therefore not of ultimate importance.

The physical body is referred to as the gross body, which,

as mentioned, is different from the self. *Bhakti* also describes the concept of the subtle body, which is also different from the self, or the soul. The subtle body consists of the mind, intelligence, and the false ego (all of our temporary, material identities). The *Bhagavad-gita As It Is* explains that the subtle body accompanies the soul from life to life in the material world, and carries with it the infinite impressions it has accumulated over numerous lifetimes. That's why we may meet someone for the first time and feel an instant connection, or pick up an instrument and immediately know how to play it, or have a bizarre experience in a dream that feels real or familiar.

A *bhakti* practitioner's journey is one of gradually trying to identify more as a soul that *has* a gross and a subtle body, as opposed to *being* the gross or the subtle body. The gross body, subtle body, and the soul all require attention in order to progress on our spiritual journey.

The gross body can be nourished with the right exercise, diet, and sleep regimen, among other things. We also need to earn a livelihood to maintain the body and its relations.

As it relates to the subtle body, we can tend to the mind through such things as meditation, good association, and being in touch with and working through our emotions. The intelligence can be fortified by things like seeking guidance, cultivating spiritual knowledge, and studying the lives of people who are wise. Examination of our false ego is also necessary in our spiritual quest. The false ego is the force that causes us to identify with our gross body, our mind, and our intelligence. By understanding our false ego, or all the worldly conceptions we have about ourself, we gain insight into our present psychophysical conditioning. When we use this insight to engage in service to the Divine, leveraging our unique strengths and talents and avoiding our pitfalls, the falsity of the ego falls away, and we identify exclusively as the soul. As an example, if you see yourself as a good parent, and a talented singer, and a holder of grudges, you can choose to teach your child how to imbibe spiritual qualities. You can sing gospel. You can explore your grudges and how they hold you back. In essence, you can start to understand more about your nature, and the strengths and limitations of your mind and body. You can explore what about yourself is perception, and what's reality. You can distinguish between the traits that are fixed, and those that you can work on. You can pray, and seek counsel. As a result, you become grounded in the temporary reality, and engage it in service of achieving the eternal reality, and begin to bridge the gap between the two.

The soul, of course, also requires careful attention. How can the soul be nourished, according to the *bhakti* tradition?

There are many ways in which a *bhakti* practitioner tries to live her life and connect to the soul, but the most important aspect of day-to-day life is the chanting of the Hare Krishna *maha-mantra* (*maha* means "great," and *mantra* means "freeing the mind"), which runs as follows: Hare Krishna, Hare Krishna, Krishna Krishna, Hare Hare/ Hare Rama, Hare Rama, Rama Rama, Hare Hare.

The *mantra*'s literal meaning is, "Oh energy of the Divine, O Divine, please engage me in your service." This *mantra* is so powerful that chanting it and sharing it is considered to be the greatest of all humanitarian activities, as it has the power to halt all types of suffering, including those caused by one's mind, by other living entities, and by the elements of nature.

According to *bhakti* philosophy, to chant this *maha-mantra* is to associate directly with God. It deepens our relationship with him, and it also helps us to develop universal spiritual qualities such as compassion and empathy. The *mantra* can be chanted quietly (yet audibly) on beads (*japa*), or in song (*kirtan*) with groups of people (*sankirtan*). There are no conditions to chant this *mantra*—anyone can chant it, at any time, under any circumstance. We can say it when we're happy, sad, angry, prayerful, hopeful, or anything in between.

The soul wants nothing more than to love, and to be loved. And to love means to serve. In fact, the meaning of *bhakti* is "devotion," and therefore the practice of *bhakti* is aimed at becoming instruments of God's compassion by being kind, truthful, and loving towards ourselves, each other, and all living beings. In this way, we are serving each other and ultimately serving God, with whom we have a personal, loving, active relationship.

The *bhakti* philosophy also places great importance on having spiritual guides, or gurus. A genuine guru is one who has deeply understood and imbibed the philosophy, and who has thus gained control of the senses. A guru is one who views him or herself as a representative of God, and who shares God's message without interpretation, self-interest, or the desire for worship. A significant rite of passage for a serious *bhakti* practitioner is to formally become the disciple of such a guru, where the disciple vows to meditate daily, and follow a specific lifestyle conducive to spiritual development. Because the guru is understood to be the representative of God, to be of service to the guru is a profound honour. The guru lovingly helps explain *bhakti* philosophy, answer philosophical questions, contextualize spiritual tenets, allay doubts, and provide a spiritual perspective to the disciple's life. It's also said that when the guru gives an instruction, it is accompanied by the empowerment to fulfill that instruction.

The *bhakti* practitioner's ultimate goal is to stop moving from body to body in the material world, and after death, to reunite with Krishna, and the feminine aspect of

God, Radha, in the spiritual world, rendering loving service (*bhakti*). Radha and Krishna eagerly await our return, but allow us to utilize our free will to have a sojourn in the material realm for as long as we desire. It's said that the soul cannot imagine the depths to which she is loved by Radha and Krishna. And so, to assist her in the journey back to the spiritual realm, Radha and Krishna send support, especially through the guru, and the *maha-mantra*. All that is required by the soul is the *desire* to return. The human form of life provides a valuable opportunity to foster that desire through spiritual activities, which will elevate our consciousness during life, and ultimately at the time of death. The consciousness at the time of death in turn determines our next destination. The Hare Krishna faith, as with many spiritual traditions, therefore outlines an ideal way to live, and an ideal way to die—one in which the devotee can try her best to remember Krishna. However, the process of dying is extremely stressful for the body and mind, and the practitioner often needs some assistance to remember Krishna.

In an ideal situation, a Hare Krishna practitioner would die hearing and/or chanting the Hare Krishna *maha-mantra*, with a drop of holy water and a *tulasi*[1] leaf on the tongue, *tulasi* beads around the neck, dust from a place of pilgrimage (often referred to as "*Vraja raj*") on the body, and sandalwood paste (*tilak* or *chandan*) on the forehead. The practitioner would have some kind of paraphernalia previously offered to the deity in the temple, such as a piece of cloth or a flower, and pictures of Krishna in the room. In the most ideal situation, the practitioner would pass away in a holy place of pilgrimage such as Vrindavan or Mayapur. Often, to help a person remember Krishna

---

1. *Tulasi* is an auspicious plant, also known as holy basil.

at the time of death, devotees will read to him from the *Bhagavad-gita As It Is*. Of all these ideal circumstances, the presence of the Hare Krishna *maha-mantra* is foremost, and sufficient on its own.

This philosophy of *bhakti*, also known as "Krishna consciousness," was brought out of India and into the western countries by a great personality named A. C. Bhaktivedanta Swami, affectionately known as "Srila Prabhupada" or "Prabhupada" for short. Known as the *founder-acharya*, or teacher, of the Hare Krishna movement, Prabhupada wrote many volumes of books and opened over a hundred temples, restaurants, and farm communities around the world in a short 12-year time span prior to his passing in 1977.

✦ ✦ ✦ ✦

A Short History of the Bhaktivedanta Hospital

In the early 1980s, four medical school students in their early 20s—Ajay Sankhe, Girish Rathod, Dhaval Dalal, and Vivek Shanbhag—felt the need to provide free, holistic care for the millions of impoverished people in their hometown of Mumbai. Each of the four young students had ample opportunity to join larger hospitals or open their own clinics, and thereby live financially sound lives. But, out of compassion for those in need, they made a conscious decision to serve the slums of Mumbai instead. And so their journey began, under the guidance of a Hare Krishna monk, Radhanath Swami. Their model was simple: they would venture out into the slums of Mumbai, lay out a little mat, sing Hare Krishna, and provide free basic healthcare to the thousands of its inhabitants. Eventually, each of the four young men married women who happened to have complementary skills (including in medicine), and their little team began to grow.

After some time, a community member donated a used ambulance, and the team rented out the ground floor of an apartment building that they converted into a clinic. Today, with the continued guidance of Radhanath Swami, they have a 300-bed hospital with state-of-the-art facilities and a holistic care model that people around the world have started to notice. They treat people holistically "from womb to tomb," with programs for everything from pregnant women and their unborn babies, to a comprehensive, world-class palliative care program for patients and families, and everything in between.

Today, the hospital relies heavily on sponsorship and fundraising and has a payment model that allows those who can, to pay for their treatments, and those who can't, to be covered as much as possible. They continue to provide free healthcare in various slums and villages throughout India.

Perhaps their most famous charitable pursuit is the annual Barsana Eye Camp, where the doctors perform free cataract surgeries to the impoverished residents of Barsana (located in the Mathura district of Uttar Pradesh), enabling people to regain their eyesight after decades of blindness.

As with all their projects, the mandate is to provide holistic care for the body, mind, and soul, based not only on modern science but also on universal spiritual principles.

꙳ ꙳ ꙳ ꙳

Holistic Care and the MATCH Guidelines

The Bhaktivedanta Hospital is not alone in recognizing the importance of holistic health. The Nursing and Midwifery Council in the UK identified the importance for their colleagues to assess each patient's physical, psychological, social, and spiritual needs. Research in the UK, Europe, and America has identified links between spiritual wellness and increased life expectancy, less pain in cancer patients, and longer survival rates following cardiac surgery.

The global rise in mental health challenges, including increasing rates of anxiety and depression, underscores the urgency of addressing well-being from multiple dimensions. Causes of anxiety and depression include loneliness, a feeling of lack of accomplishment, identification with factors beyond one's control (e. g., tying self-worth to external circumstances), and an overall lack of control (e. g., exposure to distressing news, various injustices).

Healthcare professionals around the world will agree, and I saw it vividly at the Bhaktivedanta Hospital, that each aspect of holistic health affects the others. When we are physically unhealthy, it could influence social and psychological well-being. When we are psychologically unwell, it could affect us physically. And so on.

Taking care of ourselves holistically is fundamental for everyone, because suffering is universal. The *Bhagavad-gita As It Is* states that in the material world, there is no escape from suffering, including the maladies of birth (the process itself, as well as the need to keep taking material bodies), death, old age, and disease. This is true regardless of race, nationality, religion, or any other bodily designation. At the time of death, people of every background ask the same spiritual questions (e. g., What is the purpose of life? Can I be forgiven for the things I did wrong? What happens after death? Is there a God?) and experience profound realizations and anxieties (e. g., loss of control, increased vulnerability, regrets, anxiety for the future).

The Bhaktivedanta Hospital stresses that our suffering cannot be ignored. Attention to each of the dimensions of holistic health—physical, psychological, social, and spiritual—must be addressed proactively and consistently; not only in times of crisis. By doing so, the *bhakti* texts state that we can fulfill our truest potential and ultimately halt the repetition of birth and death altogether in the material realm, and reunite with the Divine in the spiritual realm.

The foundation of holistic living at the Bhaktivedanta Hospital is captured by the acronym "MATCH." It was devised by the staff based on the writings of Srila Prabhupada. It encompasses the main principles of comprehensive wellness, common in multiple spiritual texts. Living according to the MATCH guidelines is encouraged for staff, volunteers, patients, and their families. Not fully imbibing the MATCH guidelines does not preclude anyone from practicing *bhakti* or from working at the hospital, nor does it warrant judgment from others. Rather, the guidelines provide perspective and inspiration for anyone who strives to live a holistically healthy lifestyle. The guidelines, at a high-level, are as follows:

M: Mercy

All people should be compassionate, kind, forgiving, loving, and nonviolent. Vegetarianism is encouraged to exercise compassion for animals and the earth, and for healthier living.

A merciful mindset is directly in line with the nature of the soul, and therefore brings peace of mind, a sense of alignment to one's true nature, and a deep, meaningful connection to oneself and all others.

A: Austerity

As much as we may have an aversion to the idea of austerity, like all the MATCH elements, austerity is embedded in the fabric of every genuine spiritual tradition.

Refraining from intoxication is an austerity that is

encouraged in the Hare Krishna faith and also for the patients and staff at the Bhaktivedanta Hospital. Avoidance of intoxication has positive effects on the body and the consciousness.

Additionally, austerity means to voluntarily accept inconveniences for the sake of others. According to *bhakti* texts, the soul relishes the opportunity to be of service to others, out of love. When we love someone, we automatically want to assist them. For example, if your brother is ill, you might choose to sacrifice your plans or money to help take care of him. Hopefully, he genuinely appreciates it, and that act of sacrifice could deepen your relationship, as well as his desire to reciprocate. From a *bhakti* perspective, since a practitioner's goal is to cultivate his loving relationship with God, well-conceived austerity is a way to deepen and strengthen that relationship. In every tradition, one of the most important ways to serve the Divine is to care for one another with the vision that every living being is one of his children. Holistic care models and research suggest that rendering service to others is good for our physical and mental health as well.

Austerity also means to tolerate the urges of the senses. In other words, we try our best to have self-control, rather than being controlled by our compulsions, which leads to balance and good holistic health.

T: Truthfulness

Truthfulness doesn't only mean refraining from lying and being deceitful. For those who want to imbibe this principle more fully, it also means refraining from gambling. Perhaps recreational gambling seems innocuous. But the nature of gambling subtly reinforces a mentality that can seep into the rest of life, characterized by the thrill of winning, sometimes cheating, and gaining more and more without having to earn or contribute. And, it can easily become addictive.

At worst, the World Health Organization states that gambling can lead to severe consequences, including mental illness, relationship breakdowns, family violence, illegal activity, and even suicide.[2]

To be truthful is also to take ownership and accountability for our actions. By doing so, we can foster deeper relationships and unlock exponential personal growth.

For the staff at the Bhaktivedanta Hospital, truthfulness also means to be consistently accountable, and to be honest with patients and their families. One of the biggest mistakes a caregiver can make is not telling a patient about the severity of her disease, which is commonplace in India, as a way to seemingly appease a patient.

Truthfulness requires courage. But it brings meaning by grounding us in reality. In addition, truthfulness frees us from the fear that comes when we hide from our demons, and relieves the strain of maintaining facades.

C: Cleanliness

Internal and external cleanliness is essential for holistic living. Externally, cleanliness means to bathe once or twice a day, and to regulate one's sexual relations to avoid illness, both mental and physical.

Internally, cleanliness means living with integrity, as outlined in other MATCH elements like mercy and truthfulness. It involves cultivating sincerity, good intentions, and striving to become our best selves by nurturing virtues such as peacefulness, self-control, patience, and wisdom.

By cultivating these virtues, and consciously working to remove the traits that hinder our ability to live in integrity,

---

2. https://www.who.int/news-room/fact-sheets/detail/gambling

we increasingly experience our potential, and that of others.

H: Holy Names

If Bhaktivedanta Hospital patients are open to spirituality, the staff and volunteers will encourage them to chant the names of God according to their particular beliefs. If a patient is not inclined towards spirituality, this principle won't apply for that individual, though it still inspires the hospital atmosphere and its staff.

The Holy Quran states, "And the most beautiful names belong to Allah; so call on Him by them." (7:180)

The Bible teaches us that, "He who calls upon the name of the Lord shall be saved." (Romans 10:13; Acts 2.21; Joel 2:32)

In his purport to a verse in the *Srimad Bhagavatam* (another yogic text), Srila Prabhupada states, "Any nomenclature that is meant for the Supreme Lord is as holy as the others because they are all meant for the Lord. Such holy names are as powerful as the Lord, and there is no bar for anyone in any part of the creation to chant and glorify the Lord by the particular name of the Lord as it is locally understood. They are all auspicious, and one should not distinguish such names of the Lord as material commodities." (2.1.11 purport)[3]

A connection to God through his names is a proven way to increase calmness, focus, productivity, a sense of shared humanity, and spiritual strength in a world where suffering is inevitable.

How MATCH Creates the Hospital Atmosphere

Even seasoned *bhakti* practitioners may struggle to fully imbibe the MATCH guidelines. Again, more than a set of rules, the guidelines serve to inspire and to provoke

---

[3]. Quotes from *The ABCs of Chanting The Holy Names of God*, Krsnanandini Dasi, p. 9.

thoughtful consideration. When one experiences the benefits of these principles, the appetite and ability to live them increases.

Using the MATCH guidelines, the Bhaktivedanta Hospital teaches people how to be holistically healthy by avoiding addictive activities, practicing compassion and empathy to oneself and to others, and establishing positive habits. It serves as a guide to decision-making, grounded in philosophy and reason. It connects us to the nature of the soul, which distinguishes this hospital as a unique landmark.

Throughout all the interviews I conducted, people tried to articulate what made the hospital's atmosphere so special. On the day after my arrival, I jotted down some of my own initial observations, that I would hear echoed in subsequent interviews, and that reflect some of the ways MATCH comes to life:

- Upon walking in the hospital, one can't help but be taken aback by how calm and serene the atmosphere is. It immediately feels more like a temple than a hospital. There is beautiful art on all the walls; the same art that can be found in temples. The halls smell of incense or camphor. Most of the staff wears *tilak*—sandalwood paste drawn neatly on the forehead to indicate that the body is a temple. Joyful prayers are conducted multiple times a day.
- Everyone, including the patients and their families, appears peaceful. Even in the emergency room!
- Every staff member is personal and friendly.
- Radhanath Swami has advised the staff to "be fanatic about cleanliness"—and it shows. A clean environment is a proven way to elevate the consciousness of patients

and their families. You'll not find a speck of dust anywhere at the Bhaktivedanta Hospital.

- The Hare Krishna *maha-mantra*, sung by Srila Prabhupada, is heard faintly in every corner of the hospital, including in elevators and stairwells. It's also heard in the mortuary. According to *bhakti* texts, the soul can hover near the body it just left, and can therefore benefit from hearing the *maha-mantra*.
- The meals provided are vegetarian, healthy, and wholesome.

One of the most impactful ways holistic care comes alive is through the Spiritual Care team, whose job is to tend to patients' minds and souls through establishing meaningful connection. And, if a patient is interested in spiritual knowledge, this team will share it. Even more than the doctors, this group of caregivers is trusted and loved by the patients, so much so that many of them remain in contact well after being discharged.

✤ ✤ ✤ ✤

Closing Thoughts

There are numerous reasons why the Bhaktivedanta Hospital is so special. During my time there, I found the staff to be particularly inspiring. Patients are attracted to the staff for their simplicity, humility, faithfulness, dedication, and sincere service orientation. The staff is constantly working on themselves and trying to check any vices, because they see that these things impede their ability to serve.

Another remarkable aspect of this hospital is that the doctors and staff do not experience compassion fatigue, because they are constantly being cared for. The hospital has extensive programs not just to care for its patients, but also for its staff. These programs include hours of mentorship, spiritual training, and personal and professional development courses free of charge. The leadership also provides discounted schooling for the staff's children (at their affiliated school), and in some cases, will even assist the staff in finding or financing homes. Staff members experience such an abundance of care, that they feel the need, responsibility, and inspiration to pay it forward—and this spontaneous, natural, enthusiastic mood of care is felt by all patients and their family members.

In the pages that follow, you'll read about lives changed, including my own. You'll read about patients who don't want to be discharged, and staff members who don't want to go home at the end of their work day. You'll read about first-class management from a team who has no formal management training—just heart. You'll read about care models that have the potential to make the Bhaktivedanta Hospital a global centre of excellence. You'll read stories of sorrow, triumph, love, and spirituality. My sincere hope is that these pages will at least convey some of the magic that is the Bhaktivedanta Hospital.

PART ONE

❦ ❦ ❦

Touching Ground

A journal entry upon the author's arrival at the Bhaktivedanta Hospital

Journal Entry: Arriving at the Bhaktivedanta Hospital

Radha Bhakti
January 10, 2014

The last two months in Vrindavan were everything I wanted and more. Reuniting with the children at the Sandipani Muni School was beautiful and tragic all at the same time. The last time I volunteered there, the poverty of the children broke my heart, and I felt compelled to serve them as best I could. But just a short time later, I realized that I had so much to learn and receive from these kids. They were happy without all the comforts of the West. They seemed more carefree, spiritual, and loving than any other children in the world.

There were more reunions too—my international friends returned, the locals remembered my name and little things about me (the shopkeeper remembered my favourite cookies!), and my friendships in Vrindavan grew stronger and deeper. It felt like I was home again.

Every day, I would wake up at 3:30 a.m. to attend the morning prayers and classes at the Krishna-Balarama-Mandir, which was a short walk from where I was staying. Then, I would head to the school for the day, return home for a rest, and then meet with friends for dinner and *kirtan*. Every opportunity I had, I would also visit the Radha-Damodar Temple.[1] Prabhupada used to live in this temple

---

1. "Radha" is the name of the feminine form of God. "Damodar" is another name for Krishna. In the *bhakti* tradition, we say her name before his, and therefore most temples are referred to as the "Radha-Krishna Temple," often substituting the name "Krishna" for another of his unique names, as in the "Radha-Govinda Temple." Throughout this book, there will be

before he ventured to the West, and I feel so connected to him when I sit in his rooms, which are perfectly preserved. Prabhupada called the Radha-Damodar Temple the "centre of the spiritual world," and I truly felt that while I was there. I also was able to visit the tombs of other great *bhakti* saints while in Vrindavan. I felt peaceful, grateful, and connected.

Here in Mumbai, there is a sharp contrast. I'm back in the midst of bumper-to-bumper traffic, skyscrapers, countless slums, and billboards that tell me that my skin is too dark. My heart hurts in separation from Vrindavan. But Mumbai has all the aspects of city life that I love: the lights, the buzz, the cafés, the charm, the beautiful beaches lined with enormous palm trees, and, of course, the people.

I arrived just a few days ago, and am staying in the cozy flat of my dear cousin, his wife, and their six-year-old son. They live in Bandra, which is one of the most happening areas of the city, just off Hill Road, close to the Bandra Promenade where I can sit in cafés overlooking the beach to write and people-watch. My cousin's father, my uncle, is sadly on his deathbed, and is staying close by. I will visit him whenever the family allows and is appropriate.

Tonight, I have been invited to the Bhaktivedanta Hospital for their Annual Day Celebration. I have no idea what that means, nor do I know what to expect. Dr. Komal Dalal, one of the leaders at the hospital, asked me to attend; she said it would be a good introduction to the hospital and its culture, and a nice, informal way to meet some of the staff and Trustees. Starting next week, I will go to the hospital to stay for the week. I'm petrified of living in a hospital. What will I see? What kinds of awful sounds will I hear? I really

---

many references to Radha-Krishna temples, substituting "Krishna" for one of his other names. Additionally, "Hare" is yet another way to address Radha. Saying "Hare Krishna" addresses her before addressing him.

wanted to stay here in Bandra and commute to the hospital every day, but it takes at least 1.5 hours each way, which isn't practical since I will be conducting some interviews in the early morning hours. Reluctantly, I have agreed to stay at the hospital during the week, and then come back to Bandra on the weekends. My stomach is queasy just thinking about it. But tonight will be an easy introduction to the hospital and the staff, and I will be back home in no time.

At about 5:00 p.m., I am sitting in the backseat of the car, and the family driver begins the long haul to Mira Road, where the Bhaktivedanta Hospital is located. As we arrive in the area of the hospital, we stop a few times to ask people to direct us. This looks nothing like Bandra, or anywhere else in Mumbai that I've seen. It is grey, and filled with old, dilapidated buildings. There is dust everywhere, stalls selling clothing or household items, and food vendors lining the street. We drove past a number of slums on the way here.

Soon, we arrive on Mira Road. I notice there are no animals or rickshaws; just a number of pedestrians, bicycles, and vehicles. It is not calm by any means, but it is somehow not as busy as the centre of the city either. Signs for the Bhaktivedanta Hospital are carefully and evenly placed along the divider on the road: "Care for your body, mind, and soul." When I see the signs, I feel somewhat calmer. Anything with the word "Bhaktivedanta," the title bestowed upon Prabhupada early in his devotional life, makes me feel safe and at ease.

We pull up across the street from the hospital, and I nervously walk towards the front entrance. I walk slowly past the open metal gates and a security guard. He stops me, and politely asks, "Hare Krishna, can I help you?"

"Hare Krishna, I've been invited to attend the Annual Day Celebration by Dr. Komal Dalal," I say nervously in Hindi.

As soon as I say her name, his face lights up and he gestures for me to continue.

The hospital is a beautiful pink building with a fountain and garden outside the front entrance. The festivities today are all outdoors. Men, women, and children are everywhere. They are laughing, talking, joking. I'm in the midst of a carnival, it seems. There are games for the children, prizes, tons of food, and beautiful *rangoli*[2] and other decorations everywhere on the parking lot and grassy areas outside the hospital. Everyone here is wearing *tilak* on their foreheads. The women are dressed in beautiful, colourful *saris*[3], and I am suddenly conscious of my current attire: a black Indian *kurti*[4] with dark green trousers and a black oversized scarf that I am wearing as a shawl. I feel a little out of place, but completely at home at the same time. Gratitude and excitement bubble up inside of me.

I am smiling, taking pictures, exchanging "Hare Krishnas" with the people I see. There is a makeshift wall of pictures of some of the staff filled with appreciations for the work they've done. There are pictures of doctors, janitors, and shopkeepers. Little balloons and ribbons fill in the blank spaces of the wall. It is so charming and beautifully imperfect, and it is clear that everyone here is a family.

I take my seat in a large grassy area, with many chairs facing a stage. There are reserved areas at the front, for consultants and Trustees. I sit in an empty chair towards the middle of the audience, and I take in everything around me.

In front of me is a large stage with a podium on the left,

---

2. Indian art, consisting of patterns created on the floor, made of such things as coloured rice, coloured sand, or flower petals—often seen on festive occasions.
3. A *sari* is traditional Indian dress for women.
4. A *kurti* is a long Indian-style shirt.

and the deity of Prabhupada on the right. There are also deities of Lord Jagannath (a form of Lord Krishna), as well as his brother Baladeva and sister Subhadra. These forms of Lord Krishna and his family are really special to me. They have a unique form, with enlarged eyes and mouths, outstretched arms, huge smiles, and no feet, hands, or legs. According to *bhakti-yoga* texts, Lord Krishna and his siblings took this form while hearing narrations of their childhood pastimes in Vrindavan. They were feeling such ecstasy, that their eyes got bigger and their limbs withdrew into themselves. Given their mood of complete joy, these forms of the Lord are said to be extremely kind and compassionate, eager to give blessings and love to all.

I can't believe I'm at a hospital—it feels like I am at a temple. The smell of camphor permeates the atmosphere, the sun is setting, and there are twinkle lights along the stage and lining the trees. It is an intimate atmosphere filled with a positivity I can taste.

A few moments later, the program begins. The two emcees are staff members of the hospital, and they begin by asking the entire crowd to rise and sing a prayer, entitled the *Siksastakam*, together. It is the prayer the staff chants together every day, four times a day. I stand up, baffled; I've never seen anything like this at a hospital before. After we all sit back down, the emcees begin their banter in Hindi. I can understand most, but not all of it. The crowd is loving it, laughing with abandon at their jokes. Some dances and dramas follow, and I'm genuinely impressed by the artistic talent of the staff and some of the staff's children. I look to my left, and to my shock and amazement, both Giriraj Swami and Radhanath Swami arrive. I'm floored—to be able to see both of these wonderful monks is my good fortune, and I had no idea they'd be here.

I pull my notebook out from my bag and scribble, "I feel like I'm in Vrindavan. This is a little Vrindavan miracle."

In between acts, I see Dr. Komal Dalal. She was my main point of contact while I was still in Canada. I had met her briefly in Vrindavan as well. She was there for a few days attending some lectures by Radhanath Swami. She somehow recognized me even though we had never met before. I was walking down the street after school one day, and I heard, "Radha? I don't know how I knew it was you, but I am Komal! It's so nice to meet you," and she gave me the sweetest, warmest hug. I was very grateful to have met her before coming to Mumbai.

Komal calls for me to sit with her near the front of the audience, and I do. We embrace, and I thank her for inviting me. She introduces me to a few people sitting near her, and then a panel discussion begins on the stage.

Someone named Dhaval Dalal takes the microphone, and introduces himself and three other doctors named Ajay Sankhe, Vivek Shanbhag, and Girish Rathod. The four of them founded this hospital together, and he is expressing his appreciation for each of them. His voice is gentle, just like his demeanor.

Then, Dr. Sankhe speaks. "It was October of 1995 that we laid the foundation of this hospital," he says. "We didn't have any other stone to use, so we used sandalwood, the same stone we turn into paste and mark our foreheads with. We had a *kirtan*, and we prayed for a nice hospital. Finally, in 1998, we were ready to open our doors."

Dr. Sankhe, the Managing Director and Chief Pediatrician of the hospital, is tall and thin. While his voice is soft, he has a powerful presence. He wears glasses and has a broad smile. He is dressed in a short-sleeved white button-down shirt, and brown dress pants. There is something about this man that commands respect. From his face, I can see he is kind and virtuous. The audience is silent as he speaks.

"Here we are, 16 years later, and we are so grateful to all of you for your years of service. Many of you have been with us since the beginning. You are all working tirelessly to help this hospital be successful, and remain on the platform of the heart. We are not here to make a profit—we are here to serve. We work very hard to preserve this culture, and to make sure that our collective mentality does not become one of profit mongering. This simply cannot be done without each of your loving service attitudes. Words cannot express our gratitude. This hospital is a loving offering to Prabhupada, and all of you are fulfilling this offering."

Dr. Shanbhag chimes in, "Every day we see the sacrifices you are all making, and you are all doing them with joyful hearts! You all embody compassion, which is exactly what Prabhupada would want."

"We started this hospital wanting to provide a holistic care facility based on universal spiritual principles. This is what Prabhupada wanted—for every living entity to take up spirituality, whether he is Hindu, Muslim, Jewish or Christian—it doesn't matter. If we can all learn to be good Hare Krishnas, good Christians, and so on, can you imagine the unity, the positive impact we can have on the world? If our association makes a Muslim or Christian a lover of God, this is our purpose, because only through that love can people be truly happy and united." says Dr. Rathod.

Dr. Dalal says, "Prabhupada says in the preface of the *Srimad Bhagavatam*: 'Human society, at the present moment, is not in the darkness of oblivion. It has made rapid progress in the fields of material comforts, education and economic development throughout the entire world. But there is a pinprick somewhere in the social body at large, and therefore there are large-scale quarrels, even over less important issues. There is need of a clue as to how humanity can become one in peace, friendship and prosperity with a common cause.' At our hospital, we have a common cause—to treat everybody holistically—body, mind, and soul, and to help people connect to God, if they are so inclined. We are all children of God. We are all human. We all have the same organs, the same blood. There are no divisions. Hearts can reform in a hospital, and this is necessary for there to be real peace and prosperity in this world."

Dr. Dalal is speaking so emphatically that I see people in the audience wiping tears from their eyes.

Seriously, where am I? I think to myself.

"There have been many Muslim patients who have expressed deep love and appreciation for the Bhaktivedanta Hospital," says Dr. Shanbhag. "Just today, I asked a Muslim patient why he loves our hospital so much. And he said, 'You are all Allah's people. You are truly devotees, and you've encouraged me to try to be a better Muslim. I am very grateful.' This is our success. This is what Prabhupada wanted for the world."

"Countless patients have started chanting Hare Krishna, or saying their *namaz*[5] regularly, or attending church weekly, directly as a result of having contact with the Bhaktivedanta Hospital. This is all due to your undying devotion," says Dr. Rathod.

My head is spinning with thoughts and questions. The panel continues to talk about the early days of the hospital and share inspiring patient stories.

"In the earliest days, before we even opened this hospital, we were lovingly guided by Radhanath Swami, who has been our guru, our guide, and our dearest well-wisher ever since. He has been with us from the beginning, when we

---

5. A *namaz* is an Islamic prayer.

were all just medical students. We simply would not be here without him," says Dr. Rathod. "Giriraj Swami has been a supporter of ours also from the very beginning, and has even opened our sister centre, a hospice in Vrindavan. I'd like to call both of them to the stage. Please join me in welcoming them."

The crowd erupts in applause as the two Swamis make their way to the stage.

"Hare Krishna," says Giriraj Swami, who is now standing at the podium. "It is my great honour to be speaking to you all today. The Bhaktivedanta Hospital has become a true example in holistic and palliative care. The way the management team runs it is beyond the management books; they manage with their hearts. They're not so concerned about making money."

To me, this is already clear.

"This hospital reminds me of Govardhana Hill,"[6] he continues. "This special hill in Vrindavan serves Lord Krishna and all of his friends by providing water, grass for the cows, shelter from the weather, and a playground for the Lord. What makes it so special is that the hill takes great pleasure in serving the people of Vrindavan. In the spiritual world, even a hill is animate and can express joy. If someone is begrudgingly serving you, you won't enjoy it, and you won't fully be able to appreciate it. I feel in my heart, not just as a well-wisher but also having been an observer and a patient here myself, that the staff here is in the same mood. You all just *want* to serve more and more. Whether you are mopping the floors or performing a surgery—no one is treated

---

6. In Krishna's earthly pastimes, in the midst of a devastating and torrential rainfall, Krishna, at the tender age of 7, lifted the Govardhana Hill with the pinky finger of his left hand, and it served as an umbrella for 7 days and 7 nights for all of the residents of Vrindavan. It is known to be animate, desirous to serve Krishna and his devotees.

as inferior or superior, and every single one of you has a service attitude. You have so many opportunities to go work at other hospitals that are more prestigious, where you can make more money, but you stay here because of your unparalleled mood of service. Patients who have been discharged want to continue their relationships with you because they are based on love. It is for this reason that I am confident that this hospital will always flourish, so that you can continue doing what makes you the happiest—serving. Thank you very much. I am so inspired by all of you."

I'm so swept up in this moment, that a part of me begins to wonder if I'll even want to go back to Bandra on the weekends.

Radhanath Swami then takes the microphone. Although I've only met him briefly, I have heard his lectures many times, and I have always felt deeply enlivened and inspired by them.

"I am so happy to be here with all of you tonight," he begins. "The name of this hospital is the mission of this hospital—to exemplify Prabhupada's compassion. Prabhupada was awarded the title 'Bhaktivedanta' when he became a renounced monk. He left Vrindavan to travel around the world and share spirituality out of pure, genuine compassion for all living beings. Devotees of the Lord, of all faiths, are naturally compassionate. The greatest service one can render to Lord Krishna is to experience inconvenience for the service of others. There are so many examples in our scriptures, and in all spiritual texts, of sincere devotees who sacrificed for the betterment of humanity. Lord Jesus Christ and Prophet Mohammed are two wonderful examples. Prabhupada is another perfect example. He was always concerned about our physical, psychological, social, and spiritual health. Our mission is to serve as instruments of Prabhupada's compassion.

"Over the years, this hospital has endured unimaginable challenges. There were points when it felt impossible to continue. But all of you remained united in servitude, and passed through so many obstacles. Just like Govardhana Hill—when faced with torrents of rain and devastation, it only made Govardhana Hill shine brighter. When devotees remain united, their challenges attract Krishna's grace. When the storms were coming, Krishna with his little finger, lifted Govardhana Hill, serving as an umbrella for all of Vrindavan's residents. *He shows up when we are united.*

"A grateful heart is one that is always eager to serve. The Bhaktivedanta Hospital's foundation is in devotional service. We can't love and serve humanity unless we love each other. Thank you so much for your dedication and commitment. The results speak for themselves. You are nourishing others but at the same time you are also feeling so nourished. This is real service, real satisfaction. Thank you very much."

The crowd claps, stands, wipes tears. Everyone is beaming. The emcees say a few words, and bid everyone a goodnight. The crowd begins to disperse.

My stomach is flip-flopping all over the place. I'm in the middle of nowhere. I'm still decompressing and digesting my experiences in Vrindavan. And now I'm about to live in a hospital. *This* hospital. Surrounded by sickness during the week, and then seeing my uncle on his deathbed on the weekends. I'm nervous, and uncertain. And I'm feeling a growing spark of enthusiasm to be part of something so monumental.

I'm starting to understand why Niranjana Swami wanted someone to write about this hospital. The greatness of this institution, the selfless service and sacrifice it took to build and maintain it, the struggles they've experienced along the way—it is a story that should be told.

I went from feeling excited about embarking on an adventure and writing a book, to realizing that actually, this has nothing to do with me. Somehow, I, little Radha Bhakti from Toronto, have landed in this mystical spot here on Mira Road and I get to be the instrument that tells this story. I almost don't know how I got here. But at this moment, I'm feeling like this is what I was meant to do. My whole life has led to this opportunity, right here, right now. I'm feeling so small in the greatness of this evening, this hospital, these people. A feeling of deep gratitude washes over me, and a huge sense of overwhelm.

I collect myself, say a few goodbyes, meet the family driver, and return home.

January 13, 2014

My bag is packed, and I'm all ready to move into the hospital for a week. I haven't yet gone inside the hospital (the Annual Day celebrations were entirely on the hospital lawn), and I have no idea what to expect.

I arrive at the hospital, duffel bag and laptop in tow. There is a sign right outside in Hindi that says, "Joothe math uthariye"—*"Please do not remove your shoes."*

That's weird. Why would anyone remove their shoes?

A friendly security guard lets me through. I feel like everything is happening in slow motion. I pull open the glass door, and am floored. Right in front of me is a beautiful deity of Prabhupada. The deities of Jagannath, Baladeva, and Subhadra are on a mobile altar right beside Prabhupada, and the smell of incense and camphor fills the air. There is a tray of yellow carnations in front of Prabhupada, along with a small copper vessel with water and a matching tiny spoon. To my left, there is a small book stall, carrying a number of Prabhupada's books, some pendants, CDs of devotional prayers, and magazines. Paintings of Krishna's pastimes line the walls. There are women wearing *saris* and *tilak*, and women wearing full burqas. The men are neatly dressed, many of whom are also wearing *tilak*. There is a man in a white uniform mopping the floors in front of me. It's striking how immaculate this place is. In the background, I hear the faint recording of Prabhupada singing *Hare Krishna, Hare Krishna, Krishna Krishna, Hare Hare, Hare Rama, Hare Rama, Rama Rama, Hare Hare.*

He is singing in the same melody that he used when he first arrived in the West. All Hare Krishna devotees are familiar with this very simple, yet deep rendition of the chant.

I slip off my shoes, and touch my head to the ground in front of Prabhupada to offer my respects. I use the small spoon to place a droplet of water in my right hand to wash it, and then take one of the carnations and place it beside Prabhupada's feet. I realize I am not supposed to take off my shoes, but I can't help myself—I need to remove my shoes to offer respects and a flower, as I would in any temple.

I fold my hands in prayer.

"Hare Krishna, Srila Prabhupada. I have no idea what I'm doing here."

I am struck by how peaceful the atmosphere is. I don't feel any of the apprehension I normally feel inside a hospital.

I slip my shoes back on, and follow signs for the Spiritual Care department, where I was instructed to go. Another staff member named Gopikanth greets me warmly, and takes me up five flights of stairs to my room. On the way, I see more paintings, patients and their families, drinking water stations, and I hear more of the soft chanting. I also see another janitor mopping the stairs as we climb them. There is not one speck of dust anywhere.

We reach the fifth floor, turn left, and walk down a wide

corridor. This corridor has five rooms that serve as living quarters for senior devotees, or for patient families who want to stay with their loved one for extended amounts of time. My room is #5—the last one on the left. It has two white doors that close with a sliding lock, fastened by a small gold lock. Gopikanth opens the doors for me. I step inside. Directly in front of me is a wall of windows with a view of the hospital parking lot and the road. There are two ceiling fans and an air conditioning unit on the top left of the windows—a necessity in this sunny, muggy heat. There is a sofa, a desk, a chair, and two hospital beds. There is also a small table on wheels, the kind that patients use at hospitals to eat from their beds.

There's a speaker, and Prabhupada's singing fills the room.

On the wall to my left, there is a large picture of Radha-Madhava, the main deities in Mayapur, West Bengal, an important place of pilgrimage for the Hare Krishna community. On the wall to my right, just above the sofa, is a large and beautiful picture of Prabhupada smiling. [I would later learn that this was the room Yamuna *Devi*[7] stayed in while she was very sick before she passed away. She wrote about many of the meaningful experiences she had while staying here. She was a powerful pioneer of the Hare Krishna movement, and one of Prabhupada's first disciples. This makes me feel connected to her in an indescribable way.]

I spend the day meeting with a number of the nurses in the Spiritual Care department; the true heart of the hospital. These men and women befriend each patient and learn about their lifestyles. They ask questions about their diet, sleeping habits, relationships, and learn anything else

---

7. A respectful term to use after a woman's name.

the patient is willing to share. The patients are incredibly attached to their Spiritual Care nurses, and I can see why—they are so easy to speak to, so genuine, so pure of heart. They are a powerful group of people.

I speak also with Dr. Ajay Sankhe, the Managing Director of the hospital, and we discuss the organizational processes and the fundamental challenges he faces in keeping a certain mood and culture within the hospital amidst exponential growth. I am really inspired and motivated to help as best I can.

Towards the end of the day, a Spiritual Care nurse shows me to the hospital prayer room, identical to any temple room I've ever sat in.

As I sit in this room and reflect on the task ahead of me, I feel overwhelmed. There are so many people to talk to. I want to have a tour of the hospital, understand their operations, speak to patients, families, and staff, and figure out how to structure the book. I have about a thousand questions.

Tonight, I will go to sleep with my head racing, but also feeling very much at peace.

PART TWO

❧ ❧ ❧

Breaking Ground

Interviews with two Founding Doctors and two Trustees. Note, all interviews are written in the voice of the interviewee.

Interview with Dr. Girish Rathod

Founding Doctor and Orthopedic Physician
February 3, 2014

On Medical School and Meeting the Other Founding Doctors

I don't think any one of us could have imagined that this hospital would grow into what it is today. We were just kids, trying to do something good in the world. And now I'm one of the founding doctors of this incredible institution, along with Dhaval, Ajay, and Vivek.

I first met Dhaval in 1982, as we were in the same class at Bombay University, doing our MBBS. I was drawn to him immediately—he was energetic, enthusiastic, and simple-hearted. We became friends instantly. He was also the person who introduced me to *bhakti*. He was going to the Juhu temple every Sunday with his father, and one day I decided to go with him. I never looked back. I started going regularly and also attending the events the Krishna devotees held at our university. All the devotees were so peaceful and happy, and I wanted to be a part of it.

I met Ajay at a *bhakti* get-together in Khar. My first impression of him was that he was saintly and calm, and that is still true today. I met Vivek an hour before an exam we took at the Government Law College at Churchgate. He was sitting on a lower rung of a quaint, curved metal staircase, peacefully chanting on *japa* beads, while I was frantically cramming in everything I could about HIV. I don't think we spoke so much that day, but the memory of the first time I saw him is an abiding one.

Eventually, as we were all interested in spirituality and

attending the events put on by the local Hare Krishnas at our college, the four of us came together. We soon discovered that there was a desire in our hearts to do something for the underprivileged people of Mumbai, or Bombay, as it was then called. We completed the five years of classroom training for our MBBS, and then started our mandatory year-long internships.

In 1986, we were all interning at a local hospital. It was at this time that, after getting the blessings of our seniors, the four of us founded "Hare Krishna Medicos." Our vision was to provide basic medical care in the slums of Mumbai while also sharing spirituality with our patients. In this way, we thought we could serve people's bodies, minds, and souls. It was, and still is, the vision we try to deliver—holistic care for one and all. We have always been very affected by the poverty that surrounds us. When we were young, we were so fired up—we all felt a need to help the underprivileged in some way.

Servicing the Slums

Our first official project as Hare Krishna Medicos was to go out into camps, or slums, to help people who either couldn't afford treatment or didn't have access to medical facilities due to distance or a lack of knowledge. We were doing this on top of our internships. Our very first camp was in Palghar. I remember feeling nervous and excited at the same time. We met with the *Sarpanch*[1] and introduced ourselves, and he informed the villagers that there were doctors there to provide free services. Some people thought we were frauds. I'm sure we were a bit of a peculiar sight. We stood

---

1. A *Sarpanch* is the head of a village.

there, these four young medical students with stethoscopes around our necks, and we sang Hare Krishna *kirtan* with one set of *kartals*[2] to accompany us:

Hare Krishna Hare Krishna Krishna Krishna Hare Hare
Hare Rama Hare Rama Rama Rama Hare Hare

We also had a recording of Srila Prabhupada's *kirtan* in the background when we were not chanting ourselves. At this point, we didn't have a vehicle or anything—it was just us, out in the open.

We were always welcomed with open arms because there was a severe scarcity of doctors in those rural parts. The residents of the slums accepted us very sweetly and gratefully. We used to examine them and give them free medication. We knew what to expect, that in general they were not healthy. Still, the poverty and rampant illnesses—which were preventable—affected each of us deeply. We treated people mostly for general weakness, malnourishment, and skin disease. We'd give B-complex medicines, multivitamins, cough syrups, eye-drops, and skin ointments. Most of the men living in the slums were field workers, all living in huts and other humble circumstances with their families.

We didn't have a lot of money. We were each interning and earning 750 rupees per month.[3] We'd pool that money and use it towards the camps. We were managing our own affairs, doing everything ourselves. Medical representatives would come to the hospital where we were interning and provide sample medications for the doctors' use, and the hospital would let us use those for our camps. Between the samples and our stipends, we were able to continue giving free medications. We'd also use our own money to buy med-

---

2. Hand cymbals are often used in musical meditation sessions.
3. 750 rupees is roughly $11 USD.

ical supplies. At this point, none of us was specialized; we were all doing general medicine.

We got so much joy by serving these people and sharing spirituality, and we could see that the patients were also joyful. The response was overwhelmingly positive. Hundreds of patients were coming. The world was presenting so many opportunities for us—working at various hospitals, continuing education, opening our own clinics as family physicians—but we felt that we had a responsibility to help people who simply couldn't help themselves. And we knew we had the knowledge and tools to really help people—not just their bodies, but also their minds and souls. It was our calling, and we all knew it. But we weren't sure how to move forward.

We consulted senior Hare Krishna devotees and asked them for direction. The consistent advice we'd get was to dedicate all our activities to Lord Krishna—that no matter what we did, we should do it as an offering to the Divine. They also convinced us that post-graduate studies would be beneficial, that the knowledge we'd gain could help more people in more ways. With that, we all pursued the Master of Surgery (MS) degree.

※ ※ ※ ※

A Community of Doctors Develops

Around this time, we were introduced to Radhanath Swami, and he quickly came into our lives and into our hearts. He became our guide as it related to our medical careers and even our personal lives.

It so happened that during our post-graduate degrees, we all covered the basic specialties we'd need at a hospital. I specialized in orthopedics, Dhaval in internal medicine,

Ajay in pediatrics, and Vivek in dermatology. After some time, Bimal Shah, another devotee and doctor, joined our team. He specialized in general surgery.

We all started to get married, and by some divine arrangement, some of our wives were also doctors. Ajay's wife specialized in gynecology, and Bimal's wife in anesthesia. In retrospect, I can very clearly see that this was not a coincidence. How rare it was that we all specialized in different areas, enough that we could eventually go out on our own.

While we were studying for our postgraduate degrees, it was a huge rollercoaster. We would start in the early morning, around 7 a.m., and finish by 2 a.m., at which time we'd have some dinner together. We were wondering why we were putting ourselves through all of it. It was like a being in a war zone, with constant patients, surgeries, and emergencies. At one point I went to Radhanath Swami and said, "It's practically impossible for us to continue; it's impossible for us to survive physically." In six months, I had gone from 61 kg to 44 kg.

Almost in tears, I said to him, "Being in the temple is so wonderful and peaceful! But med school and working in a hospital is so much of a struggle. There are so many politics and unhealthy competitions, and it feels like a war. I'm thinking about moving into the temple to live the life of a monk, rather than continue on this path."

The Swami very kindly looked at me and said, "Girish, it is better if you remain in a place where you can appreciate the temple, rather than stay at the temple and not appreciate it."

That became like a survival statement for me. Throughout this entire ordeal, we not only continued our camps, but we expanded them. We somehow found the time for it and, in a way, it kept me sane. It made me remember why I wanted my education—to help the impoverished. Being in the slums kept us so far removed from the desire for prestige, and from all the politics. We were just offering medical care and chanting *kirtan*. Although we were there to give, I received so much—it was so good for my peace of mind, career, and spiritual life.

We started going to different parts of Mumbai and then elsewhere in India. We'd go to the Mahalaxmi slums, Dharavi, Duktan, Lonavla, and even Rishikesh. On evenings and weekends we would seek out slums, put up our banner, and sit down and start a small *kirtan*.

We practically adopted a village in Palghar. There, we trained social health workers on such things as personal hygiene and the negative effects of alcohol. Those very health workers are still incredible counselors today. They have built a beautiful temple worth two crore[4] rupees.

Eventually, we received an ambulance as a donation. This was a huge feat for us. We used the ambulance to take us to different parts of India for camps, where we would do *kirtan*, distribute *prasadam*[5], and examine people, and some of our wives and other volunteers would act as compounders distributing medicines. This is how the wonderful journey of the Bhaktivedanta Hospital began.

✤ ✤ ✤ ✤

The Search for a Base

Some more time passed, and it became clear that we needed a place where we could station ourselves on a more permanent basis. By now, Radhanath Swami was the fibre

---

[4]. 1 crore equals ten million.
[5]. *Prasadam* translates as "mercy," and is foodstuff or articles offered to the deity.

of our existence, just like the fibre in a cloth. Every part of our life was directed and nurtured by him. He advised us to be within 1.5 hours away from the Radha-Gopinath Temple in Chowpatty. He told us to maintain a good balance between the material and spiritual, and to always ensure that we were properly taking care of ourselves and our families, so that no one would ever feel neglected. And he was very adamant that we should always work toward establishing loving relationships with each other, based on trust, affection, and mutual respect.

At first, the group didn't envision having a hospital; they envisioned a small nursing home of sorts in Palghar.

But Dhaval and I were the dreamers. When we were students, we would be in our hostel together, lying down on our beds, and we'd dream about having our own hospital or medical facility. We shared a room, and this was where we'd discuss our dreams for hours in the midst of our studying. We'd be up all night. In retrospect, I can tell you that, in the end, we received much, much more than we ever dreamed of.

As we began searching for a place to station ourselves, we carried a picture of Hanuman—the warrior god in the form of a man-like monkey—with us for good luck. Just over 500 years ago, he incarnated as Murari Gupta, who was a doctor in the time of Chaitanya Mahaprabhu.[6] We naturally had a special affinity for Hanuman. We would pray to him to inspire people to give us some land. We had no money, and would mainly approach small-time business owners, and cotton and diamond merchants. Vishakha *Mataji*[7], Dhaval's wife, would look after the fundraising.

---

6. Chaitanya Mahaprabhu (1486–1533) is Krishna himself. He incarnates as a devotee to teach the path of *bhakti-yoga*.

7. *Mataji* is a term used to address a female with respect; literally translates to "Mother."

After a long time of looking, we found a place to rent in Palghar. We were thrilled, and we started a small clinic. What a huge milestone for us! We ordered a deity of Hanuman, and we told Radhanath Swami that we were now going to have a ceremony to officially install the deity in our new facility. His response was, "This is wonderful. But don't make any permanent plans to stay at that location."

What?

We were so confused—Palghar seemed like the best place, and the response was amazing. Patients were coming nonstop. The atmosphere was nice, with chanting in the background at all times, and photographs of Srila Prabhupada everywhere. We charged patients very little.

But, under the guidance of the Swami, we kept looking.

We found a nearby nursing home that we decided we wanted to purchase. Everything was perfect. The only downside was that we were really unhappy to be so far from the Radha-Gopinath temple—it was a three-hour commute, one way. But that nursing home was ideal, just next to a metro station. Plus, it was already established. It had 35 beds, and the capacity for 35 more. It was all in a fresh, new, up and coming neighbourhood, catering to educated people. We thought this was an ideal arrangement, as we could have this nursing home and continue with the camps as well.

We brought Radhanath Swami to the facility and asked him what he thought. We were so excited, and sure that he would be pleased. He was so kind, and said it was very nice, but concluded with, "In my humble opinion, this is not a good place for you."

We were shocked. Everything was arranged; only a signature was required. All the documents, all the arrangements; everything was ready—we just had to sign.

"This is very far from Radha-Gopinath Temple, and the medical practice here is too busy. You will never have time to go to the temple. Being in this location will not be good for your Krishna consciousness," the Swami said.

We were again advised to find something within 1.5 hours of the temple. We continued with our search, hopeful that Krishna would provide the ideal venue.

Mira Road was literally the only place we did not look at first, as we thought it was just a small pocket of the city. We took Radhanath Swami, and as soon as he got there, he looked around, smiled, took a deep breath, and said, "This place has fresh air. It has an auspicious name,[8] and it is one hour from the temple."

We found a small flat close to Mira Road Station and started our first outpatient department in 1993. It was small and a bit cramped, but it was lovely. It had low ceilings, and we had two long benches outside where patients would wait for their turns. We had a long board that had the names of the doctors and their degrees. Our deity of Hanuman was right at the front. We called it Chaitanya Clinic, and it's still there now; quite a few of our consultants practice there. Our first consultations in 1993 were between 20 and 30 rupees. The response was encouraging; patients were pouring in. Of course, all the while, we were still maintaining our camps.

Then, we took another flat to start a five-bedded nursing home, which we would soon expand to twelve beds. From day one, we had the vision that we were to provide holistic care—care for the bodies, minds, and souls of all our patients. This was our intention, as inspired by Radhanath Swami.

Our parents weren't so thrilled with what we were doing.

---

[8]. "Mira" is the name of a very well-known and devout female devotee of Lord Krishna.

My parents were prepared to help me buy my own clinic and flat. Dhaval's father had some amazing plans for him in Gujarat, and Ajay's in Palghar. I asked Radhanath Swami what he thought I should do. The Swami said, "You will all be able to do very well individually in your medical practices and Krishna consciousness. But if you remain together, then you will be able to do something for which you will be remembered in history."

We happily let go of our individual plans, much to our parents' chagrin, and remained together under the guidance and care of Radhanath Swami.

Our nursing home continued to grow, and more and more patients were coming. Within about a year and half, we were overfilled.

❦ ❦ ❦ ❦

Mira Road

The land where the hospital is now located, on Mira Road, was owned by Mr. Niranjan Lal Dalmia and his partners. Mr. Dalmia was a well-known businessman and philanthropist who, together with his partners, built residential neighbourhoods with schools and hospitals for a living. They also owned the college and school across the street. They were building a community, and were actually looking for someone who could build and run a hospital. As it turned out, a wonderful *bhakti* practitioner was working as Mr. Dalmia's assistant. After quite an endeavour, we were able to secure the land.

Hrishikesh, a senior devotee of the Radha-Gopinath congregation and wealthy businessman of the Mafatlal Industries, came to know of what we wanted to do, and he funded the project. It felt like a miracle. We could really perceive that something special was happening; it was at this point that we realized we were instruments in a larger plan. It was like we took a huge leap in the sky towards the moon; we were just a small nursing home, and then suddenly we had this huge property, where we could actually build our very own hospital.

Every single aspect of this building was carefully planned with love. It's probably the first time that doctors themselves would plan the structure and design of a hospital! We were not trained in this building business. Bimal spent so much time meticulously looking after every single detail of this building. He's the head of the surgery department, and at the time he was newly married. His wife, Kalindi, is an anesthetist. They made amazing sacrifices—can you imagine, a newlywed working from 7 a.m. to 2 a.m., every day?

Bimal would go into the markets, and choose the glass, the frames, the metals, the latches, the diameter for the doorknobs—everything! And he's a doctor! He designed the layout—where the Operation Theatre, X-rays, canteen, and wards would all be; he literally designed the whole thing.

We studied the atmospheres most conducive to healing, and wanted the design to be spacious, with ample natural light and fresh air. It is unique in shape, and with a dome where the temple room would be. It was, and still is, an offering of love to Srila Prabhupada. Radhanath Swami was guiding us in every aspect; what should be done, how it should be done, the name of the hospital, where Srila Prabhupada's deity should be placed—everything.

The deity of Hanuman now sits boldly outside the Operation Theatre and Intensive Care Unit. That is the most intense area and we wanted Hanuman to be present there—to take care of the patients, their visitors, and us as well. He is still taking care of us.

Srila Prabhupada's deity is on the ground floor, right in

the centre, as per the guidance of Radhanath Swami. He told us that since we are dedicating this hospital to Srila Prabhupada, he should be right in the centre and not somewhere in a corner.

Many patients have said that they have directly perceived Srila Prabhupada governing the affairs of the hospital, even though he passed away in 1977. One Muslim patient had a dream that Prabhupada was walking around the hospital holding his cane, ensuring that things were being properly conducted. One lady who was about to deliver a baby had a dream about Srila Prabhupada telling her, "Don't worry, everything will be alright."

Every day I feel Srila Prabhupada's grace and kindness in this hospital. Prabhupada always wanted to attract people to spirituality in order to create real peace and unity in the world. The people who wouldn't normally go to a temple or church are coming here and receiving spiritual sounds, sights, scents, and food. And Prabhupada gave us his loving disciple, Radhanath Swami. Working here has made me feel that everything we have, including our abilities, is only due to the grace of Radhanath Swami and Prabhupada.

This area of Mira Road, when we acquired it, was like a swamp; no one would come here. In fact, people used to be afraid to come here. People would ask us, "Why are you taking a place that is so remote, at the end of the city?" But today, this has become a popular part of the entire area.

And something else happened that was mystical. There was a small temple in Bhayandar in a rented place, and the devotees there were looking for land for a larger temple. This was around the same time we were looking for land for a hospital. On the day we put up our "Bhaktivedanta Hospital" sign, we saw a sign right across the road that said,

"Radha-Giridhari Temple."

Can you believe it? Two different groups of Hare Krishna devotees independently set up camp just across the road from each other in this most remote location, totally coincidentally. We, as a hospital, and them, as ISKCON Mira Road. Srila Prabhupada kindly brought the temple right outside our doorstep. It was amazing.

❧ ❧ ❧ ❧

My Vision

In one sense, we live day to day. Not every patient has an ideal experience here. That is something that keeps us up at night. I pray that in the future, every single person who ever interacts with this hospital has an incredibly positive, if not transformational experience.

Of course, we want our spiritual care projects to continue to evolve, and they are, as we try to grow and build hospitals and hospices elsewhere in India.

I'd love to see many more doctors come here, get trained, and start more genuine holistic care facilities. This is much needed around the world.

Radhanath Swami gave us a beautiful vision for this place. He told us that the existence of this place depends on three things: staying together, sharing spirituality through this project, and a genuine service attitude and disposition. That's what we are attempting to do. Radhanath Swami advised us to keep spiritual care at the centre, even for each other. Our relationships have become sweeter and deeper. They go well beyond this one life; they carry forward. Our friendship has increased; we are a real family now. So many doctors and staff members have joined us. So many people—doctors, nurses, staff, patients—have embraced spirituality as a result of having contact with this hospital. It's a gradual process; it's not that they are here for one day and then become spiritual. Transformation of heart is gradual. The Swami told us to remain pure in purpose and in our hearts. That is the secret, and the reason patients feel so comfortable here.

One day, a devotee was giving out books at the Mira Road railway station, and a Muslim woman in a burqa called him over. "Hello, what are you doing?" she asked.

He said, "Hi ma'am, I am distributing books by Bhaktivedanta Swami Srila Prabhupada."

"Are you the same as the Bhaktivedanta Hospital?" she asked.

"Yes! We are from the same temple."

"Okay, please give me two books." She took two copies of *The Science of Self Realization*. She had some contact with the hospital and said she had a wonderful experience.

People's hearts are truly touched when they come here. We want everyone who comes in contact with this hospital to leave with a soft spot for Srila Prabhupada and the Hare Krishna tradition. We see everyone who comes into this hospital as Srila Prabhupada's guest, and they are taken care of accordingly. Whoever comes in this hospital doesn't come by chance; they are invited by Srila Prabhupada. It's a special place. It's clean, and there is such a spiritual atmosphere. There was a time when people would come to the entrance of the hospital and they'd remove their shoes outside because they thought it was a temple! We had to put a sign outside: 'Please do not remove your shoes.'

❧ ❧ ❧ ❧

Serving the Devotees

One of our greatest fortunes of being in this hospital is we get to serve so many senior devotees, direct disciples of Srila Prabhupada, and some of the most esteemed, spiritually elevated, and influential people in Krishna consciousness—Bhakti Tirtha Swami, Tamal Krishna Goswami, Sridhar Swami, Malati Devi Dasi, Indradyumna Swami, Niranjana Swami, Yamuna Devi Dasi, Candramauli Swami, Jayapataka Swami, Jayadvaita Swami, Kavicandra Swami, and so many more.

I remember one time there were 12 or 13 *sannyasis*[9] here at the same time. They were all sitting in the room across from this one. Radhanath Swami came and said, "Oh my goodness, there are more sannyasis here than in GBC meetings!"[10] And I would run in with *phulka rotis*[11] to serve them to eat. I remember one patient saw me and was shocked! He said, "The surgeon who is going to operate on me tomorrow is running around with hot *rotis*!" I told him, "Serving people *rotis* is my true position!"

When Mahavishnu Swami was terminally ill, the devotees took him to Nasik because that's where he did most of his missionary work. We also offered him a place in the hospice in Vrindavan, which is a very auspicious place to die according to the tradition of *bhakti*, as it is a *dhama*, or place of pilgrimage. But he sent us a message, saying, "For me, the Bhaktivedanta Hospital is a *dhama*. I'd like to give up my body there." He came, and two days later, he passed away.

There was once a guided tour of Vrindavan with Radhanath Swami. Ajay and I couldn't go as we were caught up in work. Radhanath Swami told us, "Wherever a devotee of the Divine is serving the guru in cooperation with anoth-

---

9. *Sannyasi* is the term used for a renounced monk.
10. The "GBC" is the Governing Body Commission of ISKCON.
11. Flattened bread, coming in Indican Cuisine, *phulka rotis* are those that are fresh and ready to be served.

er devotee, that place is non-different than Vrindavan."

We try to follow this instruction very purposefully. We try to cooperate with each other in loving service to our guru and Srila Prabhupada, and all the devotees. Cooperation is necessary. It is the one thing that pleases the gurus the most.

❦ ❦ ❦ ❦

Manish

One day I got a phone call from a family physician. "Do you have a place in your ICU?" I said yes. "I have a patient, Manish. He needs to be in an ICU." He was coming from Borivali, in the north-western end of Mumbai. Next to his house was another very big hospital. I said, "You can come, but that other hospital is closer, isn't it?" He said, "Manish would like to come to Bhaktivedanta."

Sure enough, he came here and was admitted in the ICU. It was just around Radhastami.[12] He had lung failure, heart failure, and kidney failure, and he was immediately put on a ventilator. It turned out, my wife Shyamarani was acquainted with him from years before. Within a few days of arriving here at the Bhaktivedanta Hospital, Manish passed away. When he passed, there was chanting going on, Srila Prabhupada's *kirtan* was in the background, there was a *tulasi* leaf and Ganga water in his mouth, *chandan* on his face, and he was wearing a flower garland from the deity. He never practiced *bhakti-yoga* in his life, yet he had such an ideal passing.

Maharashtrians have a custom that when a body is about to be taken to the fire pyre, they tie some food to the person's wrist. It's like sending the soul off with some food for his journey to his next destination. Not only did Manish

---

12. Radhastami refers to the appearance day of Srimati Radharani, or "Radha," the feminine aspect of God.

pass away with all of the auspicious materials present, but Shyamarani also tied Radharani's *mahaprasad*[13] around his wrist. On Radhastami day, a few days before Manish passed away, Shyamarani went to the Radha-Gopinath temple. She never asks for *mahaprasad*, but somehow that day, she did. The priest gave her some *mahaprasad* that was located next to the deity of Radharani's feet. They were *laddus*, a very popular Indian sweet. She brought the *laddus* here, and that was what she tied to Manish's wrist.

Shyamarani and I were marveling at how fortunate Manish was. We thought to ourselves that Manish wasn't the kind of person who was deep into spirituality, nor was he trying to cultivate his relationship with God. And yet Krishna arranged for such a spiritual departure for him. Then we realized that at a certain point in his life, Manish had a pharmacy, and he allowed Srila Prabhupada's books to be distributed at his shop. He kept those books on his front case and table. For that one little service, we can see that Srila Prabhupada remembered him, and took care of him at the time of death. We understood that Prabhupada remembers and appreciates every small act of service one does to help bring others closer to spirituality. We understood how *alive* he continues to be. This gave me a little more faith that yes, maybe there is some hope for me, and for everyone. Prabhupada was the ideal guru, really helping his disciples and grand-disciples to come closer to the Divine. And he always reciprocates with even the smallest service.

Our faith in Prabhupada increases greatly working here. We see so often that patients pass away just as soon as devotees are available to chant for them for their last few moments. When you see patterns like this, you begin to realize that it is personal, and divine. It's happening on pur-

---

13. Foodstuffs from the plate of the deity are termed *mahaprasad*.

pose, by Prabhupada's design.

❧ ❧ ❧ ❧

Faith in Gurus

The most wonderful thing in the world is the care of the guru. His or her blessings can empower anyone. That's how we are here. Radhanath Swami, our guru, had a vision, and Srila Prabhupada had a vision. Srila Prabhupada had a vision for every living entity. In fact, all we have to do is hold onto the blessings of the guru, and everything will be taken care of. Our vision was so small, so tiny in comparison to what was given to us.

If somebody asks me what I want to take away from this place, it's easy: the memory of serving so many great souls here. There was a time when we had to close the hospital for a while. During that time, we were not thinking about the quantity of surgeries we did, or patients we saw. Dhaval and I were thinking how fortunate we were to have been able to serve such exalted people. Niranjana Swami said, "Generally everybody is more than reluctant to come to a hospital and more than eager to leave. But here I am more than eager to come and now after my treatment I am more than reluctant to leave!"

This place is more than a hospital. It is Prabhupada's home, and we're just servants helping to run it smoothly. It is well beyond me and my colleagues—we have merely been instruments to execute Radhanath Swami's plan. And he gives all credit to Srila Prabhupada, without whom this hospital would never exist. I am deeply grateful.

Interview with Ram Maheshvari

Trustee
December 12, 2014

I moved to Mumbai after completing my undergraduate degree in Commerce in Ashok Nagar, Madhya Pradesh in 1978. I moved in with my brother, Mahaprabhu Das, who was practicing law. In early 1977, shortly after my father had passed away, my brother had started frequenting the local Hare Krishna temple at Juhu, and I would go with him once in a while.

In the early 1980s, Mahaprabhu started having devotees at his house once a week for *kirtan*, philosophical discussion, and a sumptuous meal of Krishna-*prasadam*. I attended every week. Even now, 35 years later, this event is continuing and I still attend, together with my wife and kids. This was the place where I met more devotees, and where I really began to understand and appreciate the philosophy of *bhakti*. This event became quite well known and visiting monks would come often.

❧ ❧ ❧ ❧

Ever Smile Property

When the doctors were looking for land for a hospital in the mid-'90s, they were searching near the outskirts of Mumbai. My boss, Mr. Dalmia, was a builder and was aware of what they were trying to do. He was very supportive. I started working for him in 1989, after spending some time working in a cement company as a sales executive, and working in imports. Mr. Dalmia had two partners: Mofatraj and

Goenka, both reputed builders in India. The three of them formed a company called "Ever Smile Property Limited." I wasn't working for the company; I was working directly for Mr. Dalmia in his paper plant. I was looking after a bit of everything—finance, purchases, administration, and sales. He had interest in several other businesses, including developers and builders. I worked with him for 25 years.

Dalmia, Mofatraj and Goenka came together to build a residential area, and it is now known as the Sristi Complex, here in the Mira Road area. It spans about 150 acres; maybe more because there is marshy land that they cannot yet develop. As it related to the project of building a residential area, Mr. Dalmia had asked me to attend many meetings on his behalf. Under his direction, along with that of his partners, about 50 apartment buildings in this area were built and sold. While we were discussing the potential for this massive project, we came to learn about government requirements for housing colonies. The municipality had designated areas where we needed to build a college, a school, and a hospital. One of Ever Smile Property's partners built a high school. Another started Royal College, which is right next door, as well as a Muslim college which is one of the best in this area. The trio was contemplating who they could commission to build a hospital.

This was in the early '90s. At this time, the Chaitanya Clinic was already in existence. I was closely associated with the founding doctors of this hospital and I knew they were trying to build a hospital, but I didn't think this area was what they were looking for; I thought maybe they were looking for something smaller and more manageable, like a larger clinic or a very small hospital. I also wasn't sure if Mr. Dalmia and his partners would want to trust a group of Hare Krishna doctors with such a massive endeavour.

I spoke to Hrishikesh about it. Hrishikesh is a successful businessman who knew the founding doctors and Radhanath Swami very well. I told him that there was a place at Mira Road already earmarked for a hospital, and that I'd be able to initiate talks with Mr. Dalmia and his partners if that's what he wanted. It just so happened that at around the same time, Radhanath Swami was accompanying the doctors in searching for land for their new hospital. As fate would have it, the Swami had already seen this area of land at Mira Road, not knowing it was available and that it was already earmarked for a hospital, and had expressed interest. After discussing this at length with Hrishikesh, the doctors, and Radhanath Swami, everyone agreed that I should bring it up to Mr. Dalmia.

I remember one incident very specifically. The founding doctors, some other friends, and I were all in one room discussing how we could go about building a hospital, and after some time, we all left the room except for the Swami. He called me back in just a moment later, gave me some *mahaprasad*, and said, "May Srila Prabhupada empower you to accomplish this task." I never forgot that. Radhanath Swami never met with Mr. Dalmia to discuss business matters; he only ever spoke to him on a personal level, leaving everything else to Srila Prabhupada and to Krishna.

It took us three years to convince all three partners of Ever Smile Property to let us take on this project. Mr. Dalmia was the first to be convinced. He loved me like a son, and I loved him like a father. But it was actually Hrishikesh who convinced him after meeting him a few times.

Hrishikesh comes from a respected and well-connected business-oriented family, and he told Mr. Dalmia that he himself would raise or provide the funds to take care of all the building costs. Mr. Dalmia had faith and confidence in him. The other two partners took some time to be convinced, but eventually they were, primarily because they appreciated the charitable spirit of the doctors.

When, after three years, we finally received ownership of the land, I sent a one-liner to Radhanath Swami: "By your blessings, all is fine." His response was also short: "On behalf of Srila Prabhupada, all blessings to you for accomplishing this."

Hrishikesh took on most of the expenses for the construction and other initial variables. We also approached some other people for help, like our friend Dr. Narendra Desai, his brother-in-law, and also a Mr. Bagaria, who was Mr. Dalmia's broker. Mr. Dalmia convinced him that this was a worthy cause and that his money would be well-utilized. Mr. Bagaria had a significant amount of money he was looking to donate, so he gave part to an eye hospital, some to a *goshala*[14], and some to us. We later heavily fundraised, but initially I don't believe any major donations came from anyone else.

By this time, Mr. Dalmia had become a good friend of the local Radha-Gopinath Temple in Chowpatty. If I recall correctly, he had sponsored our Barsana Eye Camp, a camp where the doctors annually perform free cataract surgery for the impoverished residents. I took him there once, and I remember he had tears in his eyes when he met people who thought they were blind but could then see again, and all because of a group of doctors who operated on them for free.

As the story goes, we were able to build the hospital. Today the Bhaktivedanta Hospital is a well-oiled machine, running on universal spiritual principles under the expert

---

14. Cows are housed in a *goshala*.

guidance and loving care of Radhanath Swami. What a journey it was to get here!

I am continuously inspired when I think about Radhanath Swami. He never thought about making a hospital—he thought only about how he could best serve his spiritual teacher, Srila Prabhupada.

Srila Prabhupada was never after profits. He always said that we should just serve people, and then the money for maintenance would come. Radhanath Swami, from the very beginning, said that the ideal is that every person who walks into this hospital should get the best treatment possible, and pay whatever he or she likes. We're not quite there yet, but we're hopeful. Earlier we were always in the red. Now, we break even.

❦ ❦ ❦ ❦

A Spirit of Giving

One of the many unique things about this organization is that truly, we are only in the business of giving. The goal is always to pay as much as we can for patients. We believe that the more we give, the more people will feel inspired to give back. Our constant meditation, inspired by Radhanath Swami, is to provide selfless service. The rest will come.

Interview with Hrishikesh Mafatlal

Trustee
December 16, 2014

Early Days

My wife and I became *bhakti* practitioners soon after we got married. We had our first daughter in 1978, our second in '85, and our son in '87. I joined my family business after graduating and training for two years. In 1993, I completed an Advanced Management Program at Harvard.

I am currently the Chairman of our business group; it's a fourth-generation family organization. We are named after my father, Arvind Mafatlal, and operate primarily in chemicals and textiles. We have three public companies that are all independent. I am the Chairman of the three companies; two chemical and one textile. I enjoy being the Executive Chairman, as it gives me the flexibility and time to dedicate to the hospital and temple activities.

My older sister Maithili Priya and her husband Dr. Narendra Desai were the ones who introduced me to Krishna consciousness. They were both great devotees. In fact, my brother-in-law had actually met Srila Prabhupada. They started having get-togethers with devotees at their home in the early '80s and they would always invite me and my wife, Radha Priya, to attend. We would go occasionally, but it wasn't really a priority for us. Then, our family went through some major difficulties, and that became the catalyst for us to prioritize spirituality much more. We began going to the Juhu temple, which was the only Hare Krishna temple in Mumbai at the time. It was there that I had the privilege of meeting quite a few wonderful and senior devotees like Giriraj Swami, Gopal Krishna Goswami, and

Purnapragya *Prabhu*.[15] All these people made a huge impression on us. We were so inspired, and also surprised that we felt that way, because we had always assumed that spiritual life was only for elderly people, and my wife and I were only about 31.

My father was a devout spiritualist. A lot of saintly people would come to our home while we were growing up. I respected all of them, but I never felt particularly inspired. But being at the Juhu temple was a very different experience. Radha Priya and I were meeting 20-year-olds who were so bright, and who discussed the philosophy in such an attractive, practical way. They were completely committed to their spiritual practice, and not fanatic. They were grounded, and relatable.

❦ ❦ ❦

Meeting Four Young Aspiring Doctors and Devotees

The get-togethers in people's homes were increasing steadily, both in frequency and in number of attendees. My wife and I started going regularly, and we would see Ajay, Girish, Vivek, and Dhaval, who were in the process of completing their pre-med degrees. They were the original four founders of the hospital.

We all became good friends. It was so inspiring for me to see these young, unmarried doctors so committed to providing free healthcare to the underprivileged. They had many opportunities for their careers, but they chose to share their interests in medicine and spirituality with others. They began with going into the slums of Mumbai to

---

15. Using *Prabhu* is a polite, and respectful way to address someone.

offer some basic healthcare, and later expanded into their Barsana Eye Camps. To this day, the hospital continues to offer free healthcare in various slums in India, and every year they go to Barsana to perform free cataract surgeries. In the beginning, they did everything on their own. The whole group would go on weekends to provide healthcare, *kirtan*, and meals to a number of patients. They did the nursing, the examinations, the cataract operations, the cooking—everything.

They were motivated simply by the desire to stay together, to do something good, and to please their spiritual guide, Radhanath Swami. I was not a medical man; I was a businessman. It was amazing for me to see that their need for money was secondary.

I was a friend and well-wisher, and I would also help financially. The costs weren't so big at that time—the team would travel by the local trains and they'd also pitch in from the stipends they were receiving from their internships. Our relationships were strong because everyone was sincere, and we were all trying to practice the Hare Krishna faith together. The more time we spent together, the more our admiration for each other grew.

❦ ❦ ❦

The Vision for a Hospital

As a financier, I was heavily involved when we started to look for land for a hospital. It took some time, but we came to know that Ram's boss was a big builder. As it happened, they were building a whole residential complex and had a space that was specifically meant for a medical establishment. The land was officially ours in 1994. It was a huge feat. Prior to obtaining the land, we had the realization that none of us had any idea how to run a hospital. So for a few years in the early 90s, we took up a contract to run a floundering hospital in a suburb north of Mumbai called Virar. That was an exceptional experience for us. We got exposure in all facets of the organization—understanding the costs, hiring people, recruitment, patient care—everything. This hospital was experiencing some financial difficulties, and we were contracted to help them break even and increase their occupancy level. I wasn't directly involved in the management; it was the doctors who were dealing with the daily affairs of the hospital. I met with them regularly to bring in my experience from a business perspective. I'd look at their income and expenditures to help them make ends meet. It was a joint effort.

It took us almost three years to build the Bhaktivedanta Hospital. Initially, the budget was going to be within eight crores. Somehow, we were able to arrange the funds, but by the time we did, the cost had grown to ten crores. We ended up using the assets that were already built to get a loan for the additional two crores, which we knew we'd be able to pay back within a couple of years.

Dr. Bimal Shah, a surgeon, was the doctor who spearheaded the entire effort of coordinating and guiding the architect and the contractor. He is a top-notch surgeon, but he took real interest and care in the construction of the hospital. Whatever Dr. Shah takes on, he does with great attention to detail. We had a top-tier architect firm, VOLTAS, a Tata company, and a reputed contractor working with us.

A very senior executive from my company was overseeing the entire project. The contractor was Mr. Ramesh Dalal, who had handled many multi-crore projects before. He actually donated half of the fees back to the hospital, because he believed so much in what we were doing.

We had planned to open the hospital in 1996 for Srila

Prabhupada's centennial, but we were a little late. Finally, in January of 1998, we opened our doors. It was so much larger than we ever expected; we didn't know how we'd manage on a day-to-day basis.

※ ※ ※ ※

Early Challenges and a Focus on Spiritual Care

It wasn't without struggle in the beginning. In 2003, we had some serious labour issues. A union was formed, and the situation became extremely hostile, even though it was only a handful of people who were causing the upheaval. We decided to close the hospital for a year. That was a tough decision. We made sure to take care of the several hundred people—doctors, nurses, and others—who were innocently forced to stop working at this time. We paid them every month for the full year. Everything but the clinic was closed, and even the founding doctors were unsure of their own future.

We met with Radhanath Swami to brief him on the situation every time he was in town. He never really asked about the minute details of the dispute, but in 2003 during the closure, he gave us one instruction that changed everything.

He told us that we had to refocus. We had recently put tremendous effort in reinvigorating spiritual care, but we were still struggling to just manage the hospital and recoup our costs. We still were not focused enough on what was meant to be the *heart* of the hospital—spiritual care, with a charity focus. That instruction enabled us to realize that we had become too absorbed in the nitty gritty and we almost forgot that we built this to be, first and foremost, a spiritual and holistic care institution, and not a profit-making entity.

So, with Dr. Ajay Sankhe at the helm, we put extra

strength behind the Spiritual Care department and ensured that the right mood—one of love, trust, and care, was in every fibre of the hospital's being. And that included raising funds to pay the unionized employees more, so they felt more valued. Eventually, we raised enough, the union withdrew, and we were able to reopen our doors.

That was a major chapter in our history that taught us that we need to maintain our relentless focus on spiritual care, and not on profits. Our desire is to help, serve, and relate to people as emotional, complex beings. Everything else—the equipment, the contracts, the numbers—is all incidental.

Ajay's leadership was at that time, and continues to be, beyond exemplary. He is very humble, and everyone gravitates towards him. He actually comes from a farmer's family; his parents lived in a village a couple of hours away from the hospital. He relates very well with every staff member, many of whom also come from villages. He is a very fair leader. It's not a technique—he's just straightforward and real. His open-door policy, the way he dresses, the way he speaks—it's all very genuine. He's calm, especially in crisis or when there might be reason to panic. He is so comfortable talking to the housekeeping staff or the nurses; he is relatable and kind to everyone. They all talk to him about their personal problems. He's a Director, but he doesn't act elitist or entitled. His leadership really got us through the labour dispute and helped turn everything around.

Initially, there were some Hare Krishna devotees who had some apprehension about us opening a hospital. They were concerned that perhaps this was a project that was placing too much emphasis on the body, rather than the soul. The soul, according to our scriptural texts, is our real identity. The disapproval from some fellow *bhakti* practitioners was disappointing and difficult for us to deal with, but Radhanath Swami continued to comfort and encourage us. There was one statement he made at the opening of the hospital in 1998 that none of us ever forgot. He told us that this hospital will successfully help people become more spiritual through our holistic care model. It will eventually turn out to be one of the biggest and best ways to share *bhakti* and overall spirituality with the masses. There were moments when it was hard for us to believe; moments when we were really struggling. But now, we have hundreds of thousands of patients coming in and so many programs that help people enhance both their health and spiritual lives. We've seen that spiritual care is not just a remedy; it's also the prevention of future disease.

Caring for One Another

We want to serve everyone associated with us, including our staff. Mira Road is very far in the suburbs, and difficult to get to. We bought a number of flats in the neighbourhood, and staff can rent them or stay for free depending on the situation. We have also provided loans to staff members.

Real estate prices in Mumbai have multiplied by five or six times in the last several years, so we try to do our best to see that our staff is comfortably situated. There is, of course, a professional relationship, but at the same time, we try to help them if they have any other anxieties like large debts or family issues. We have a counsellor system for emotional support, which is so important for everyone, especially the doctors and nurses. Doctors and nurses can obviously feel emotionally affected by the physical trauma they see regularly. It is important that they have a counsellor to speak to. Otherwise, they could easily become indifferent or allow other issues to crop up. We want all our patients to feel deeply, wholly cared for by our medical staff, and for this to happen, the staff needs an outlet. They have to be well situated. So, we try our best to take care of our staff holistically as well.

❦ ❦ ❦ ❦

Daily Care

In the service industry, organizations like airlines, banks, and hotels all say that the "customer is king." They train their employees well, and they in turn provide high levels of service and friendliness. But, often times it's a technique; it's not necessarily from the heart. The moment an employee is "off-duty," they're switched off.

Here, the doctors and staff care for their patients with their hearts, and it truly touches people. When there is a sick child and the doctors lovingly leave their homes to care for the child and comfort the parents, imagine the impact it has. No matter caste, creed, or religion, loving care is given to anyone and everyone. This is the culture that Srila Prabhupada would want, and this is always the goal.

Patients are very open to spirituality. In India especially, doctors are respected, and their opinions are taken very seriously. When our doctors suggest spirituality as a branch of holistic care and as a means for having a healthy life, patients are very receptive. It is during times of sickness that people begin to question life and seek solutions to their problems beyond their physical ailments.

In our experience, cancer patients are especially open to spirituality. They experience a plethora of emotions. All of them have questions about the existence of God and their purpose in life. We are planning on building a cancer department over the next few years.[16] For now, we have a cancer surgeon, Venu Madhava, who treats patients in the hospital and goes to rural camps multiple times a week.

❧ ❧ ❧ ❧

Today and Beyond

I am now a Trustee. I help ensure that all the broad parameters on which the hospital runs are being met. There are some that are common to all hospitals and some that are unique to ours. We always concern ourselves with spiritual care, patient experience, financial performance, and future goals. The larger principles are the spiritual ones.

We have plans to construct a new building that will cost 700 million Rupees [approx. $8.4 million USD].[17] It's worth the investment; the more people we can help, the more we will consider ourselves successful. We have seen how our holistic care model helps patients, their families, and our staff. In my experience, we have a loving, caring, peaceful atmosphere not found elsewhere.

The type of care we offer in the camps and at the hospital is attractive to everyone, regardless of religion or background. Actually, Giriraj Swami's family, who happens to be Jewish, donated $1 million for the ophthalmology department.

In those beginning days, we had no idea what we were doing. We were just living day by day. Now I look back and the dots connect. When the polyclinic was there, we didn't see anything beyond it. The hospital was supposed to be simple, but somehow it all just happened. Over the years, a lot of effort has been expended on developing our vision, and

---

16. This department is now built and fully operational.
17. This three-floor building is now constructed, as an attachment to the existing hospital.

we revisit it from time to time. But we never foresaw it in the beginning. Srila Prabhupada definitely did. Radhanath Swami did. But we didn't.

As Radhanath Swami told us all those years ago, as long as we keep the right focus, the right goal—to provide loving spiritual, holistic care—then everything will continue nicely.

Interview with Dr. Ajay Sankhe

Founding Doctor and Pediatrician
February 3, 2014

Being a Director for this project is the privilege of a lifetime. I'm not a trained manager. I'm just doing what is needed and people here are kind enough to tolerate me. In every situation, I just think, "What would Prabhupada do? What would Radhanath Swami do?"

I have a common-sense management understanding. I like to keep in touch with all strata of people in the hospital and I like to inspire or encourage them to do better. It is a top priority to keep the mood spiritual and service-oriented.

I feel that everyone here is a Director, and everyone should make decisions as such. I tell people this is their family business—we are all connected by Srila Prabhupada, and so we are all owners. As owners, they'll think differently. If they see themselves only as a sweeper, or a nurse, or a doctor, then they will just do their part and leave. But if they see themselves as owners, they might be a little more careful, or do a little extra.

❀ ❀ ❀ ❀

Spiritual Care

We have three primary goals:

1. Everyone here has an occupation with the purpose to please the Divine. One person may be a nurse, another a doctor, another a member of the housekeeping staff. We want everyone to feel inspired to serve according to their nature. In Sanskrit, this is called *Varnashrama*.[18]

---

18. *Varnashrama* is a central concept in *bhakti-yoga*, stating that one should engage in service to the Divine according to one's nature and stage of life.

2. Everyone's goal should be to genuinely serve all those who come in contact with the hospital—staff, patients, doctors, everyone. We see everyone as a spirit soul, eternally connected to God, and therefore we strive to serve them with humility. In Sanskrit, this is called *Vaishnava seva*.[19]

3. We strive to help people connect with their higher natures by sharing spirituality. We call this *Vaishnava dharma prachar*.[20]

We are not perfect and there's still work to do to ensure every visitor has a great impression of our hospital. But we believe that by keeping these three spiritual principles at the heart of our efforts, we can leave a deep and lasting impact.

In the world of medicine today, success is very much tied to profits. Every hospital has fully developed marketing teams in an effort to provide care but also for economic prestige. Here, at the Bhaktivedanta Hospital, we have no marketing department, but people are coming here loyally. That means that spirituality has its own marketing value and its own economic benefits.

When we first opened the hospital, there was no dedicated Spiritual Care department. The whole hospital was trying to embed spiritual care into their daily work, but we were all so busy that no one really focused on developing the department. Spiritual care in those days was the spiritual music and chanting in the background, and the offering of blessed food, but there was no focused spiritual care for patients. After a year and a half of operations, Radhanath Swami asked me how I was feeling, and I expressed my

---

19. A *Vaisnava* is a servant of God. *Seva* means service.
20. Sharing the calling of the soul (to connect with one's loving relationship with God).

dissatisfaction to him. He encouraged me to refocus on spiritual care, and put some thought into how to further develop it. By his inspiration, we divided spiritual care into categories—patients, doctors, staff, and the community at large. I created a short two-page document on how to give spiritual care to each group, and that is the basis of what you see now.

Today, the Spiritual Care department is the heart of the whole hospital.

PART THREE

❧ ❧ ❧

On the Ground

Author's personal journal entries, and interviews with the staff and patients of the Bhaktivedanta Hospital. Note, all interviews are written in the voice of the interviewee.

Interview with Chetna (Patient) and Bhavin (Husband) Rao

December 17, 2014

Chetna: No one could ever have prepared me for the moment I discovered that I had a lump in my left breast. It was earlier this year, and it took me completely by surprise. I went to my doctor at a hospital in a different part of town to get it checked out, and had a sonogram. There, they discovered that I had a large tumour. They asked me to come in for an FNAC test.[1]

I was definitely shaken, but somehow I still couldn't allow myself to imagine that I could have cancer. I was convinced that the tumour would be benign. It had to be. Cancer doesn't run in my family, I've lived a relatively healthy life, and my life was so busy—I had no time to even think of having any health issues, what to speak of cancer.

At the suggestion of a friend, we made an appointment with the Bhaktivedanta Hospital for the removal of tissue from my breast. As the appointment neared, I became more and more nervous. The c-word would pop up in my mind and I'd quickly brush it aside. But it didn't go away. I told my husband, who supported me with loving and reassuring words. We decided we wouldn't tell our son or our parents—we didn't want to worry them.

After what felt like an eternity, we arrived at the Bhaktivedanta Hospital for the tissue-removal appointment, and learned that Dr. Sunitha Prasad in the Pathology Department would perform the procedure. I had so many

---

1. A Fine Needle Aspiration, used to remove breast tissue or fluid to check for cancer cells.

questions—how does one remove the tissue? Would it hurt? Dr. Prasad was very kind and sweet, and spent a lot of time answering my questions. She made me feel comfortable both with her calming words and her gentle technique. I felt reassured and at ease in her care. She removed the tissue and I felt no pain. This was in July of this year. It was just the beginning.

The test results arrived eight days later. I didn't pick up the report; my husband did. The report suggested that it could be cancer, but that a biopsy would be required to know for sure. My husband couldn't bring himself to tell me. Dr. Prasad told us to see Dr. Vishnu Agarwal for further diagnosis and treatment. My husband said we had to go to this doctor for further consultation, but he didn't tell me why. I came to know that Dr. Agarwal was an oncologist—I didn't even know what that meant. I checked online, and learned that an oncologist is a cancer doctor. My heart sank.

We met him, and he immediately took me for a biopsy. When we arrived at the Operation Theatre, there were beautiful pictures of Lord Krishna and his pastimes on every wall. Our family is Hindu, which is different from *bhakti*, but we also believe in Lord Krishna. Seeing all the pictures of Krishna was such a pleasing sight for my eyes.

While the doctor was injecting me, this lovely Hare Krishna music was on. The doctor himself was also chanting quietly along with the music. He was chanting, and concentrating, and like that he performed the biopsy. At first I thought it was peculiar that the doctor was chanting—but in the end, it almost felt like a sacred sound bath. It felt healing. Throughout the procedure, I wasn't aware of what was happening. But in an inexplicable way, I felt calm. I mean, he was about to inject me with something like a gun and remove some tissue, but I felt comfortable in his care.

Suddenly the doctor told me it was over. I didn't even realize when it had started. "Can I get up now?" I asked him.

"Of course! Go have a nice evening with your family," he said.

He gave me some painkillers to take for five days, and said he'd get the report after eight days or so. I hate that about the medical system. Eight days before you know if you have the ugly c-word! Eight days to pretend like everything is okay, when inside, I was crumbling.

After exactly eight days we came back, and the doctor confirmed our biggest fear: I had breast cancer. The doctor told me I'd have to go in for a further PET Scan to assess what stage I was in. My husband was beside me, and began to cry. I was dazed, angry, and in disbelief. My first thought was my family. I love them so much. My husband, my son. In that moment I tried not to cry—I thought I needed to be strong for my family.

We came home that night, and didn't know what to do. We were reluctant to tell everyone. My father-in-law has a heart condition, and we were concerned about how he'd take the news. My mother-in-law also has some health issues, but we knew we had to tell her. After everyone finished dinner, my father-in-law went to sleep, and my son went to study in another room. We sat my mother-in-law down and told her the news. She started to cry. "What's the next step?" she asked. We told her we had to do a further scan. We told her we were afraid to tell my father-in-law, but she said she would tell him and that it would be okay.

Two days later, we went to a different hospital for a PET scan, and to get a second opinion. I was terrified and again didn't know what to expect. I conjured all my willpower and went. It was scary, and this hospital really felt like a hospital. Bhaktivedanta Hospital was warm and homey.

Even the patients there seemed peaceful. But at this hospital, they weren't. Everyone looked miserable. The doctors weren't harsh or shrewd, but they were extremely transactional. Here, at Bhaktivedanta Hospital, even if I'm just coordinating an appointment with administrative staff, or dealing with a nurse, I don't feel like a patient. I'm more at ease. The environment over there was too scary for me.

Bhavin: We have been to a few different hospitals. For the most part, they were fine, and people were friendly. But for us, there is just no comparison to Bhaktivedanta Hospital. Here, we are treated like family; it's not transactional at all. The staff genuinely cares for the patient, and we felt that from day one with our interactions with Dr. Prasad.

Chetna: The ambiance makes a huge difference to a patient. There is something peaceful about this entire building. The staff assures us that they are with us every step of the way, and they are. This gives me so much more strength.

The PET scan from the other hospital confirmed that I am in the initial stages of breast cancer. Since the tumour was quite big, I was told I'd have to undergo chemotherapy before going through surgery.

That was the moment I cried, more than I ever knew I could. I just broke down and released all that was pent up since this journey began.

We returned to the Bhaktivedanta Hospital, and were introduced to Dr. Nirmal Raut, the onco physician here. He is extremely compassionate and loving in every interaction we have with him. He told me that I'd have to go through a nine-cycle process of chemo, in which they wanted to monitor the tumour, and see that it would reduce. He told me to come in every week for chemo. He said it would be a long procedure, and that it could affect the functioning of the nerves.

I had so many emotions. Shock, anger, sadness. On one hand, I wanted to proceed with bravery and courage, and show my son that his mother is strong and would be okay. I didn't want him to feel like he had to take care of me—it's my job to take care of him. On the other hand, I felt overwhelmed, exhausted, and afraid.

Soon after the cancer diagnosis was confirmed, we told our son. I was feeling guilty because he's in the 12th grade, which is a crucial year for him. He'll soon have to decide what profession he wants to pursue, and I didn't want him to worry about me. But my goodness, his response was so relieving to me. More than his words, it was his grounded and reassuring energy that spoke volumes. He said, "Mom, don't worry. Science is so much more advanced now, more than ever before. Go through the treatment and everything will be fine." I told him that I was worried that he'd be worried about me. And his response was, "Mom, nothing will happen. I will pray, and my prayers won't go unheard." I'm just in awe of my son.

When I told my parents, they were understandably distraught. But they and my parents-in-law have given me so much moral support. Everyone continues to encourage me to move forward, to fight this. And they are always with me, every step of the way. I can't tell you how much strength this gives me.

Every chemo session was really difficult—I had a lot of nausea and vomiting. My hand was swollen. My taste buds were affected; I couldn't eat properly. My blood count would go down after every bout of chemo, so I had to have three injections to bring up my blood count.

Whenever I came for chemo, I met Ratikeli *Mataji* and Santosh *Prabhu* from the Spiritual Care department. They are like mentors to me. They kept guiding me, and they gave me a lot of spiritual reading material like the *Bhagavad-gita As It Is*, and *Back to Godhead Magazine*. I had a *Bhagavad-gita As It Is* at home but was always too busy to read it. But here, I started reading these books and also the *Ramayana*. My chemo sessions would last almost all day. Delving deeper into spirituality gave me more willpower, and mental and physical strength. One thing I realized is that bodily problems are just that—they are just related to the body. I had to conquer my mind. I used to feel angry, but now I can say I'm peaceful. I can't believe it's my cancer that made me feel peaceful. Growing up and even as an adult, I had so much anxiety because I used to get teased and ridiculed often. But now, it simply does not affect me. I feel compassion for people who say hurtful things. They're just ignorant. The mentoring I've received here has helped me tremendously.

That's the thing about cancer and chemotherapy. It can cause a person to lose faith in God, or it can create the deepest faith in God. And that's what happened to me. I never questioned God's existence, but in a remarkable way, the chemotherapy brought such intense suffering that I found myself praying and surrendering more, and it made me feel even closer to God. Like even though I was suffering, he was with me. The Spiritual Care team helped me feel his presence more than I ever have.

My chemo also made me have some understanding of what I read in the Gita, about not being the body. I really felt trapped inside my body. Like inside, I'm full of energy, and zest. I'm not this body that is falling apart.

Eventually the tumour shrunk enough for me to proceed with an hour-long surgery here at Bhaktivedanta Hospital. My husband was just outside, waiting for me, alone. When I was being wheeled into the OT, I was scared. But then

I looked at all the pictures of Krishna, and I submitted myself. I said to him, "You are around me, and you are within me, so I submit myself. Whatever is meant to happen will happen and I know you will take care of me and my family."

Ultimately, I had to have breast removal surgery, which took place a couple of months ago. I was very calm. In fact, I could see that even Bhavin was quite calm. The parents were all crying, badly. When I was being taken in, I said to them, "You relax, I'm happy. I'm going to be fine." I wasn't crying. I knew everything would be okay. I had complete faith in God, and I knew I was in the hands of a doctor who was very spiritually sound.

I was in the OT from 8 a.m. to 12 p.m. The surgery was about 2.5 hours, and then they kept me under observation for some time. Since that surgery, I have been feeling better and in better spirits. I am going through the last stages of chemo now. The last chemo will be in January. In February, I will begin radiation for 25 days. The tumour was 6.5 cm.

I don't know what's going to happen. We are very much in the thick of our journey.

When I was healthy and working, my routine was so busy. My prayer regimen was very mechanical. I'd say a little prayer in the morning, go to the office, come back, check on my son, and pray again for a few minutes before bed. But I didn't read the scriptures or go deep. I didn't submit myself to God. I submitted myself after I fell ill. This disease has made me want to get closer to him. I've realized that all reversals in life are blessings, and opportunities to come closer to God, and truly surrender. Because of my cancer, I feel mentally and spiritually stronger. And my newfound spirituality has given me peace of mind, even amid my physical suffering. And now I really feel God gave me this disease because he loves me and wants me to feel closer to him, and I do. I used to care so much about having "things." But now, I'm experiencing something higher —a real higher, spiritual feeling. And it wouldn't have happened without this cancer.

My biggest support, though, is sitting right here, in front of me. My husband sees to it that I'm always adhering to my schedule for food and medicines. He runs all the errands, and he looks after us financially. I used to contribute to the family financially, but now the entire burden is on him. He's doing everything so amazingly. I can say he's my biggest support. I used to wake up early and tend to the house but now he lets me sleep and does everything himself. He says to me, "You rest. Look after yourself. Beat this cancer because we both love and need you very much."

I have started writing about my life and my disease. Ratikeli told me that I could publish it in the hospital magazine. I have a strong desire to help people who are going through this. The people at Bhaktivedanta Hospital have helped me so much. I am thankful to God that he gave me such good people, and that he brought me to this particular hospital. We didn't have this feeling anywhere else—this feeling that we will be well taken care of. I mean, I was dumbfounded when the doctor did my biopsy and I didn't even know when he started! I was just listening to him and suddenly it was just done.

Bhavin: The patient gets partially healed just by being in this atmosphere.

Chetna: After becoming a patient here, we moved to Mira Road. We had never even been in this area before, but now it is home. Whenever I'm here at the hospital, Santosh and Ratikeli spend significant amounts of time with me. They make my heart lighter. I don't know what will happen, but I really feel that I will be okay. I'm not scared. I come here happily, and I leave happily. I feel protected here. And I have the support of a wonderful husband and son. I will be okay, no matter what.

Interview with Rajesh Kadam

Manager, Spiritual Care
January 22, 2014

Before joining the Bhaktivedanta Hospital, I was in the Air Force in the National Defense Academy for three years. I was withdrawn on medical grounds and was desperate to find another job. My father was on the verge of retirement, and my sister was soon to be married. Our current residence was being provided by my father's company, and now that he was about to retire, we had to look for a new place to live.

One day in 1995, I bumped into my best friend from high school after not having seen him for 15 years. He was a completely different person! He went from being my fellow prankster—more accurately, he was the victim of many of my pranks—to a true gentleman with an abundance of knowledge. He was calm, grounded, and peaceful. I was envious.

"There is a peacefulness about you now. What's your secret?" I asked.

In response, he took me to the Radha-Gopinath Temple in Chowpatty. I heard a class from a devotee named Gauranga *Prabhu*, and I became immediately attracted to Krishna conscious philosophy. I am really drawn to discipline and cleanliness; these qualities were highly valued in the military, and they were values I really respected and tried my hardest to imbibe. I saw the same values present in the Hare Krishna tradition, but now, instead of implementing that value system out of fear, it was being implemented with love.

I started going to the temple a little more regularly with

my wife and soon became involved in the theatrical performances the devotees would put together for festivals. This is how I met Vivek, one of the founding doctors of the hospital. We acted in a play together and became fast friends, and he invited me to the Barsana Eye Camps, just to witness what was going on there.

I went, and that was it. My heart was stolen in those camps.

I started attending lectures by Radhanath Swami, and he'd use words like "humility," "compassion," and "discipline." I didn't feel I could live by these words, but I was definitely inspired by them. In 1997, I went to Vrindavan for a few days to attend a tour led by Radhanath Swami, and there, I saw that he really walks his talk. I don't know how else to explain it, but I really fell in love with him on that trip. In 2000, I officially became his disciple.

His association and example inspired me to serve more at the Barsana Eye Camps. What a privilege to serve the residents of Barsana, who are considered to be so very dear to Lord Krishna! I served at the Eye Camps for many years. I'm not a medical man, so I would distribute food, make hot water in the wee morning hours for the doctors, do crowd control, and run errands. I'd take leave from my office and go to the camp for a month.

☘ ☘ ☘ ☘

Changing My Direction

After a few years of volunteering at the Barsana Eye Camp, my father became quite ill, and it was soon apparent that he was going to pass away. I was devastated. Dr. Ashok Shetty and his wife Premlila both came to my home and read the entire second chapter of the *Bhagavad-gita As It Is* to him. They also brought all the paraphernalia that should be on the patient's body at the time of death. They changed the whole room into a temple—the walls and even the ceiling had pictures of Lord Krishna and Srila Prabhupada, so that wherever my dad would look, he would see spiritual images.

We were able to go to Vrindavan five days before he passed away because of the help of the devotees. My father was bedridden, but after discussing it with the doctors, we were able to take him to Vrindavan by train. My father was able to see the most auspicious places like Radha-kund and Shyama-kund, and we circumambulated Barsana and Govardhana Hill, and the deity of Srila Prabhupada.[2]

In Vrindavan, the devotees took constant care of my father, keeping him company and talking to him about spirituality. And it was due to the incredible friendships he had formed at the hospital that he had started chanting 16 rounds[3] of the Hare Krishna *maha-mantra* daily, and had done so for two years.

My father, in this way, had a glorious passing. It was the ideal way for a *bhakti* practitioner to die.

When I saw the personal and loving spiritual care that my father was given, I became convinced that I wanted to serve this hospital for the rest of my life, so I could pay that love forward.

I've been here now for ten years; joining this hospital was the best decision I've ever made. All my talents are put to

---

2. Circumambulation of places of pilgrimages or deities is considered extremely auspicious in the *bhakti* tradition.

3. One "round" consists of chanting the Hare Krishna *mantra* on each bead of a necklace containing 108 beads. 16 is the recommended amount of rounds for a serious practitioner, taking approximately two hours in total.

use here, and all my desires are fulfilled. I love to council, give classes, and interact with patients. It doesn't even feel like a job.

Now, I work in the Spiritual Care department as a Manager, and I report to Dr. Shanbhag. This department is very dynamic. Professional hierarchies don't really exist. We're all brothers and sisters, working together. This culture is very much encouraged by Dr. Sankhe; he insists that we all run the department together.

❧ ❧ ❧ ❧

Dimensions of Spiritual Care

Spiritual Care has four dimensions: patient care, staff care, education and training, and outreach.

Patient Care

We, as a Spiritual Care team, try to meet every patient who walks through our doors, and we try to gauge their emotional well-being. We look for symptoms of satisfaction, gratitude, humility, and joy. We ask about the patient's spirituality—"Do you consider yourself a spiritual person? Are you open to becoming more spiritual?" We are careful not to impose spirituality on anyone. If someone does not want spiritual care, we simply befriend him and make sure he feels happy and cared for. If a patient is open to it, we will speak more about spirituality and religion. Regardless, we are there just to talk. There is so much emotion for a patient, no matter what he is in the hospital for. It's nice to have someone to talk to.

We make a real effort to build a genuine relationship with each patient. They usually have questions about health or lifestyle habits, and sometimes talk about personal problems, most often regarding relationships and household life. Often, people ask for proper counselling and we try to serve them in this way. Every day, I have on average one to three spiritual counselling sessions.

Once the patient has been discharged, we invite him or her to come back after a month to attend a spiritual program put on by a particular department, depending on the type of treatment the patient came for, such as ophthalmology. The doctor will speak on a particular topic, like the best way to take care of the eyes, and then the second topic will be spiritual, like "Real Vision." We call this program the *Premanjali* Program.

We also have our *Parivatan* program for those patients who express more interest in spirituality. This is a group that discusses spiritual psychology based on the *Bhagavad-gita As It Is*. *Parivatan* means "change"—this program attempts to bring positive change to the patients' lives through spirituality.

Staff Care

For us to have strong patient care, we need staff members who are well-oriented and trained on the basics of universal spiritual principles.

Interested staff members can participate in our *Jagruti* program on Wednesday mornings. At 6 a.m., we come together and chant our *japa, tasbih*[4], or rosary until 7:30 a.m. At that time, we have a class on a verse from the *Srimad Bhagavatam*, usually conducted by Shyamananda *Prabhu*. We do a similar program on Tuesday evenings as well.

Staff can also participate in our *Maitri* program, a system that matches staff members with a "buddy" in the organiza-

---

4. *Tasbih* is a form of meditation in the Islamic tradition, where practitioners utter a glorification of Allah on each bead of a necklace.

tion. The "buddy" is someone senior, specifically associated with a junior staff member so that the latter could have someone to informally talk to about anything they'd like, whether it has to do with work or not. This has worked well for us. The mood here is very family-oriented; it's easy for people to open up to one another. We are trying to cultivate a very Vedic[5] culture.

I also like to conduct spiritual competitions. I'll write down a question, and post it on all of the floors of the hospital along with a clue as to where to find the answer, typically in the *Gita*. Of course, if someone wants to respond based on the Quran or the Bible, that's perfectly fine too. So on a particular day or week, all the staff is reading about the same topic from their scripture. It's quite fun and encourages them to read. We get about 150 participants every time.

Education and Training

The Bhaktivedanta Hospital has its own Nursing School, where we offer a BSc as well as the Registered General Nursing and Midwifery Program. What makes us unique, however, is that we also offer a Spiritual Care module. Based on the *Bhagavad-gita* As It Is, we cover topics like "Who am I?" "Does God Exist?" and "Why Do Bad Things Happen to Good People?" We also cover "Qualities of a Spiritual Caregiver," "Time Management," "Counselling Skills," "Listening Skills," and "Compassionate Communication." We are constantly adding new chapters, like "The Importance of Forgiveness," and "Special Spiritual Care: ICU Trauma, Babies, End of Life." We also provide a certificate in Spiritual Care.

---

5. This refers to the ancient Indic culture of *bhakti*, characterized by kindness, respect, and honesty.

Outreach

One of the defining principles of the hospital is the dedication and commitment to provide free healthcare to the less fortunate. Our Community Health Services group remains focused on servicing the slums of Mumbai and elsewhere. If people require more sophisticated care than can be provided in a camp, then we bring them here. Cataract operations are a common example. We'll bring someone in from a camp, along with a caregiver or family member, and take care of the costs for their stay, meals, and the operation itself. Around 60% of the cataract operations we do here are free of cost.

Everyone who comes in from a camp receives spiritual care as well. We invite them to sessions, offer them prayer beads, and offer them free *Bhagavad-gitas*.

We also have our regular Barsana Eye Camps. There, we do free cataract operations, and we offer five types of spiritual activities: 1) Continuous *kirtan* for 12 hours at a time; 2) Blessed meals; 3) We bring the deities of Radha-Gopinath and Srila Prabhupada for all to see; 4) *Yatra* (pilgrimage); and 5) Spiritual ceremonies.

After the Barsana Eye Camp is completed, we take all the staff and volunteers who participated on a spiritual pilgrimage. Patients, doctors, nurses, and relatives join us on regular *yatras* around India. We typically do two *yatras* a year, each for 4-5 days.

One of the most effective and vibrant outreach programs we have is the Bhaktivedanta Youth Foundation. We reach out to high schools and universities to get kids involved in giving back to their communities. For example, December 1 is World AIDS Day. For a couple of weeks before and after that day, we give a number of seminars in schools and colleges about education and prevention of teenage pregnancy and STDs. We speak to about 10,000 students through this program, elucidating everything from healthy relationships and the merits of celibacy to the ABCD formula: Association, Books, Character Building, and Diet. Many school principals appreciate our work very deeply and have praised us publicly.

The Bhaktivedanta Youth Foundation also has a project called "Plant a Smile." The youth involved in the foundation spend time at old age homes and with destitute people with no families simply to offer companionship. The youngsters go and talk, play games, sing songs, and just breathe youthful energy into their lives. The youth in the foundation are so inspiring—they are passionate about issues like poverty, the environment, and politics. It's a joy to work with them and help them channel their passions in positive ways.

※ ※ ※ ※

Kushal

The story of one patient, Kushal Chauhan, to me, exemplifies the power of spiritual care. He was a blacksmith with severe health issues. He was married with three children, and his wife was illiterate. He felt a lot of pressure at home to earn money, as his wife Preeti was very insecure about her illiteracy and refused to obtain an education. Unfortunately, Kushal developed a growth in his rectum that became so enlarged that he could no longer evacuate. He was bedridden with a catheter bag. Kushal was devastated, frustrated, and humiliated, and said that he would rather die than continue to live like that.

Our Health Forum workers, who are social workers, were able to help a little by paying off bills and buying food. But the more help he received, the more Kushal felt dejected. He felt like a burden, a parasite. This is, unfortunately, a very common attitude amongst Indians; they will suffer quietly so as not to feel like a burden to others. It's very hard for Indian people to ask for help. Kushal used to speak with me often. He wanted to give back to society, and expressed remorse that he was unable to contribute to the world, what to speak of his own family.

One day we were speaking, and I said, "Why don't you offer a *Bhagavad-gita As It Is* course for your neighbours?"

"It's not possible. Who would come here to be around such a sick person?" he said.

"Why not? If you'd like, I'll come and facilitate the course myself," I said.

It was as if Kushal felt a renewed sense of purpose. "Go clean your rooms!" he said to his sons. "Go tell all the neighbours we are hosting a *Bhagavad-gita As It Is* class. We'll start it tomorrow and go for three days."

Members of the Spiritual Care team arranged everything. We brought *prasadam*, and we arranged the space so that it was comfortable and conducive to learning.

The neighbours all came, and while Kushal was lying down in his bed, we all sat next to him and discussed the philosophy of the *Bhagavad-gita As It Is*. Honestly, this whole class was basically for him. I couldn't tell him that he is the soul, and not his body, as he wasn't ready to hear that message while in such pain. But being able to host a class in his home made him feel like he had purpose, like he was helping others. He listened very attentively. He heard about death, *karma*, and the soul—topics he may not have been interested in otherwise.

The class went on for three days. On the fourth day, I went back to visit him, and he started to ask me questions about death, how to prepare, and the proper way to die. He was a

Hindu his whole life, but didn't really practice any devotion. He didn't have much philosophical knowledge. He learned a little when he was a child, but then he moved to Mumbai and forgot everything. He was very proud of being born in a *brahmana*[6] family, but later realized that the title "*brahmana*" is properly acquired due to one's quality and work, not one's family. He became so humble, and so inquisitive. He developed a deep respect for the *Bhagavad-gita As It Is* and asked many questions about its author, Srila Prabhupada.

After some time, he told me that his health crisis was in many ways a blessing. He went from believing that God is cruel to truly experiencing God's love. It was amazing to see this transformation. Earlier he was only speaking of his piteous condition and feelings of helplessness, but later he really began to see everything from a spiritual perspective.

The Healthcare Forum workers were simultaneously trying to prepare Preeti to stand on her own two feet. They gave her a job, but after the first day she panicked and decided not to return. They helped her find another one, but the same thing happened. The third job they helped her find was the one that stuck. She was hired to put the labels on the back of denim trousers. She liked it. She was bringing in 3,000 rupees per month, which was quite a good amount for her family.

Kushal's eldest son, at that time in the sixth grade, was avoiding him. When Kushal became bedridden, he was pressuring his son to drop out of school and start working to support the family. We convinced him to let his son stay in school so that he could get a good job afterwards. He and his son started to develop a better relationship after that.

---

6. A *brahmana* is the highest caste in India's caste system, defined by those with a scholarly nature.

It was heartbreaking to watch Preeti deal with Kushal's illness. It was becoming more and more apparent that Kushal wasn't going to live much longer, but Preeti was convinced that feeding her husband sumptuous meals would allow him to regain his health. Kushal felt frustrated with her attempts, even though they came from a loving place, and it would cause them to argue. We explained to Preeti that he had just a few months left, and that she should prepare for that. Of course, Kushal knew he was in the process of dying as well. A few days after that conversation, Preeti was much more supportive in the ways Kushal needed, and their relationship became peaceful.

Kushal passed after Preeti had been settled in her job for about two months, and the kids were also well situated.

Kushal was able to leave his body with a spiritual understanding of life and death, and confident that his family would be okay.

It is such an honour to be involved in cases like this. Experiences like this truly make us realize that we are just instruments in a greater plan, and it is indescribably humbling to take part in a family's journey as they watch a loved one pass away.

※ ※ ※ ※

Arundhati

Arundhati Anand was another memorable patient for me. She was a policeman's wife with two children—an 11-year-old daughter, and a young son of about six. She had no connection to her other family members. While she was suffering through the final stage of cancer, her husband passed away. She was living in a mortgaged house and was in severe financial debt. I can't even imagine the anxiety she was experiencing, knowing that she, too, was soon to pass away.

Our Bhaktivedanta Health Forum Workers contacted the press, making a public plea for some financial assistance for this family. Arundhati became a heroine. So many people wanted to help her and her family. We raised Rs. 7-9 lakhs.[7] She passed away about six years ago, and even today her kids are being financially taken care of by the funds raised by Bhaktivedanta Hospital.

After the coverage in the papers, we approached the principal of the kids' school, who agreed to make their education free until the 10th grade. With this information and the newspaper clipping, we approached a bank, who then agreed to waive the entire loan for her mortgage. As soon as the kids are 18, the house will belong to them.

While Arundhati was alive, our Spiritual Care team provided as much support as they could. They were visiting her regularly, counselling and guiding. They'd even help with the cooking, cleaning, and tutoring of the children.

This is our approach—first and foremost, we try to relieve the patient of physical pain, then social, mental, and finally we address their spiritual needs. We try to treat all our patients and their families as though they were our families, too. The care we give is straight from the heart.

---

7. One lakh is Rs. 100,000.

A Dying Wish

There was once a small boy—let's call him Prashant. When he was a child, he walked into the Radha-Gopinath Temple with his family, where Radhanath Swami was visiting. The Swami took the young boy on his lap and fed him a cookie. After that, the family occasionally visited the temple, but very sporadically, and soon their visits stopped completely.

About 15 years later, Prashant was a young adult, and he became interested in spirituality. He started frequenting the Juhu temple, chanting Hare Krishna, and reading the *Bhagavad-gita As It Is*. But after a short while, he became busy with his career and stopped chanting, reading, or going to the temple.

Some more time passed, and Prashant was diagnosed with cancer. Around the same time, he received a book called *The Journey Home*, the autobiography of Radhanath Swami. Prashant loved this book, and soon realized that this book was written by the same Swami he had met all those years ago as a child. He went to the Juhu temple to see if the Swami was there, but alas, he wasn't.

Prashant came here to Bhaktivedanta Hospital to be treated for his cancer. When he discovered that this hospital was Radhanath Swami's labour of love, he was excited beyond words. He asked me, "Is he here? Can I meet this Swami?" I thought it was very sweet that he didn't realize the kind of travel schedule the Swami has, and that he's not always accessible.

"I'm not even sure if he's in India!" I said. "But let me see what I can find out for you."

"I really feel that this man is my guru," Prashant said. "I

must meet him!"

The next morning, the first thing Prashant said to me was, "Did you find him? Is he here?"

"Not yet," I said. "I'll ask some more people today."

For the next few days, he would repeatedly ask me if the Swami was here, and every day he asked if he could formally ask him to accept him as his disciple in an official *diksa*[8] ceremony.

"That's so nice that you feel he is your guru. There is a long process to take *diksa* from him. Usually it's about a five-year waiting period." I said.

Prashant was visibly disappointed. My heart went out to him, and I tried hard to locate the Swami. Finally, I was informed that he was, in fact, in Mumbai. It was unbelievable. There was one devotee who was assisting the Swami with managing his schedule, and I asked him if he could come to the hospital briefly, just to connect once with this patient. I explained the whole situation. Unfortunately, the devotee told me that the Swami's schedule was too tight, and that it wouldn't be possible. He didn't even give the message to the Swami. I tried calling the devotee again and asked if the Swami could come the next day. The devotee told me that the next day, the Swami was scheduled to leave Mumbai for Pune.

---

8. "Diksa" is a ceremony wherein a spiritual teacher and a *bhakti* practitioner accept each other as guru and disciple. At a *diska* ceremony, the disciple agrees to chant 16 rounds of the Hare Krishna *mantra* daily, and follow a set of "regulative principles of freedom" (e. g., refraining from intoxication and eating meat). At the time of *diksa*, the guru gives the disciple a new spiritual name. *Diksa* is considered to be a rite of passage for the serious *bhakti-yoga* practitioner. While it is not a requirement on the path of *bhakti*, it is considered a very happy, auspicious, and blessed occasion and accomplishment.

I was so frustrated for Prashant. In fact, it's not often that we are in the same city as Radhanath Swami, due to his intense travel schedule. I told Prashant that we should both pray for a meeting to somehow take place.

The next day, the Swami's plan was to go to an appointment, and then to drive to Pune. As scheduled, he went to his appointment, but then he told his driver, "We're not going to Pune yet. Let's go to the Bhaktivedanta Hospital."

The devotees were bewildered. We got a call that Radhanath Swami was coming, as he wanted to visit Yamuna *Devi*, a godsister of his who was a patient at the hospital at the time. He came, and spent a good amount of time speaking with her. As he was leaving her room, it was just me standing there—no one else. He smiled his beautiful smile—the one that makes me feel so loved—and then he gave me his unique warm embrace. It's the kind of embrace that just makes one feel so loved.

"Radhanath Swami, I know you're very busy, but there is one patient here who has read your book, and he has literally days left to live. He'd really love to meet you, and he considers you to be his guru. Do you think you could …"

"Where is he? Let us go see him," said the Swami.

Immediately, I took him to the ward where Prashant was staying, while all the other devotees observed and wondered where we were going. We walked into Prashant's room, and he was astonished! He just couldn't believe his eyes. He got off his bed, and bowed his head down to the floor to offer his obeisance to the Swami. Along with him, his IV stand dropped with a bang! I immediately picked up the IV stand, and Prashant began crying profusely.

"Swami, thank you so much for visiting me," he said. "Please, give me your grace."

The Swami smiled. "I'm very happy to meet you. How

can I serve you? You want *diksa?*"

Prashant very humbly looked down and said, "Oh … I'm not qualified. I can't chant 16 rounds of the Hare Krishna *mantra* because of the pain in my stomach. I'm managing about three rounds daily."

The Swami looked so kindly at Prashant, and without hesitation, he said, "I can see how sincere you are, and I will give you *diksa* right now. Your new name is Govinda Prema."

I was stunned; I had never seen the Swami give *diksa* like this before. It's such a process these days—the standards are quite high. You need to be recommended by a counsellor, you need to have chanted 16 rounds daily for a few years, and more. But that day, he initiated Prashant with so much love, and without any of those prerequisites.

Govinda Prema was baffled. He looked at me and said, "Did he just say he'll give me *diksa?*"

"He already has!" I said with so much joy. Govinda Prema was gobsmacked.

Radhanath Swami spoke with him for a few minutes, and then he departed. I walked him to his car, and when I came back to Govinda Prema's room, he was sitting and chanting.

"I have received *diksa*," he said. "I must chant 16 rounds." It was painful for him to sit for long, but he was determined. I was so inspired.

The next day, he said to me, "Do you think I can go to Vrindavan?"

I started laughing out loud. What a spiritually demanding and rich person! I admired his determination to see a holy place of pilgrimage before passing away, and his willingness to travel in his condition.

"If your desire is strong, maybe it will happen!" I said. But truthfully, I was perplexed. How would we pull that off?

I decided to write down his story, and I sent it to everyone I knew. This email went viral. It was forwarded to people around the world! One man saw my email and arranged first-class tickets for Govinda Prema to fly from Mumbai to Delhi with one caregiver. From Delhi, a car would be arranged to take us to Vrindavan.

We went to the airport, all ready to go. But when we got there, the airline informed us that due to his severe condition, Govinda Prema couldn't travel without a medical certificate. We did everything we could and called everyone we could think of, but we were defeated. I was kicking myself.

For some reason, right at that moment, I realized that on the way to the airport, we had forgotten to sing the prayers to Lord Nrisimhadeva.[9] I never drive without first singing those prayers. So I gathered a number of people, even the airport authorities, and I said, "Please, let's just sing this prayer together." We all sang this beautiful song:

> *namas te narasimhaya*
> *prahladahlada-dayine*
> *hirannyakasipor vaksah-*
> *sila-tanka-nakhalaye*
>
> *ito nrsimhah parato nrsimho*
> *yato yato yami tato nrsimhah*
> *bahir nrrsimho hrdaye nrsimho*
> *nrsimham adim saranam prapadye*
>
> *tava kara-kamala-vare nakham adbhuta-sringam*
> *dalita-hiranyakasipu-tanu-bhringam*
> *keshava dhrita-narahari-rupa jaya jagadisha hare*

At the end of the prayers, I opened my eyes, and I couldn't

---

9. A form of Lord Krishna who offers all protection to his devotees.

believe what I saw. Bhakti Charu Swami[10] was standing right in front of me! I told the Swami everything about Govinda Prema, and what we were trying to do. Very confidently, the Swami gave me the garlands that the deities of Radha and Krishna were wearing at the temple that day, and he said, "Just trust Krishna. Everything will be fine. I have a feeling you will go to Vrindavan today."

A few minutes later, the captain of the aircraft came out. The man who had purchased the air tickets for us had called a friend with some influence with the airline. His friend somehow called the captain directly and pleaded our case. The captain approached us, saw Govinda Prema lying down, and said, "If this man can sit for the whole flight, I will take him."

With utmost determination, Govinda Prema sat in his wheelchair.

"Okay," the captain said after a minute. "I'll take him."

Everyone in the crowd erupted in cheers and tears. And he went! He actually made it to Vrindavan, to such a holy place of pilgrimage. The same person who had spoken to the captain arranged for our return trip as well. Shortly after we returned, Govinda Prema passed away at the Bhaktivedanta Hospital while we were chanting the Nrisimhadeva prayers, and all the right circumstances were met.

ॐ ॐ ॐ ॐ

Staying Steady and Grounded

People sometimes ask me how I can stay unaffected and unemotional while working at a hospital. The reality is, I can't. I am affected by what I see and experience. But I feel

---

10. A prominent renunciant and guru in the Hare Krishna tradition, and a disciple of Srila Prabhupada.

that this is part of my spiritual advancement. When people cry, you cry along with them. It's an expression of love for those in pain. This job makes you go through severe sadness and intense happiness on a regular basis. Radhanath Swami says that the measure of spiritual advancement is the extent to which we empathize with others.

It's the kindness of my guru and Srila Prabhupada that by associating with the people in this hospital, I can see everything in life from a spiritual perspective. Working here trains us on all the concepts we read about in the scriptures. We always learn and read that we are not these bodies, that there is so much suffering in the material world—we are confronted with these facts regularly. Working at the hospital has truly increased my faith, and there is nowhere else I'd rather be. The Bhaktivedanta Hospital is my biggest source of happiness and inspiration.

Interview with Vineeta, Prashob, and Kamal
Palliative Care Team
January 23, 2014

The Palliative Care team provides care for terminally ill patients, either at the hospital or at the patient's home. At the time of this interview, the team consisted of three staff members: Vineeta (a medical doctor), Prashob (a psychotherapist), and Kamal (a nurse). The Palliative Care team provides an invaluable service, creating and implementing a model for which the Bhaktivedanta Hospital has become well known. In order for me to get a feel for the Palliative Care Team, the group kindly invited me to spend the day with them, accompanying them on home visits with patients and their families. Before leaving to meet patients, we all had lunch together in the hospital canteen, where the following conversation took place. A volunteer from the Youth Foundation, Ridwan, also joined us on this day. —RB

Vineeta: I joined Bhaktivedanta Hospital in 2007, and the Palliative Care team in 2008. When I joined the hospital, I participated in an onboarding program, where they thoroughly covered palliative care. This immediately piqued my interest, mostly because working in palliative care presents a unique opportunity to really talk to and befriend patients, while simultaneously using my medical abilities. I used to work as an assistant surgeon. In that role, there wasn't the same opportunity to connect with patients. It was the main reason I was feeling dissatisfied. I know this sounds funny to say as a doctor, but I really feel that love is the most effective medicine. I've seen patients heal faster with less medicine and more love and support. By working in palliative care in this hospital, I'd be able to practice *bhakti-yoga*, literally defined as the yoga of love, while also earning my daily bread. I have been a *bhakti* practitioner, or Hare Krishna devotee, since 2005. For me, this opportunity was perfect. To be able to give people some spirituality at the time of death, to help them see the role of a higher and superior existence, and to help patients and their families be a little peaceful during this most heart wrenching time, is the greatest honour.

When I was trying to become a surgeon, I didn't get into a post-graduate program. This deeply saddened me, and I fell into a bit of a depression. I went to the Radha-Rasabihari temple in Juhu, and I was praying to Krishna, asking him why this happened, and feeling lost about what to do. I decided to attend a course at the temple, and through studying Srila Prabhupada's books, I learned so much about *bhakti* and felt so inspired. It lifted me out of my depression—I realized there was so much I could do with my life, even if it wasn't surgery. There was so much more I could do as a doctor. This experience changed everything; this course taught me that there is a higher purpose and value to life. I suddenly felt, once again, that my life could be valuable.

So, when I heard about the Palliative Care department and the types of services they do, I felt it was where I should be. It felt like a calling.

Prashob: The practice of palliative care is holistic, in that we not only address the physical aspect of care, but also the psychological, emotional, and spiritual pain of the patient. We deal with patients who are in the terminal, or incurable phase of their lives. Most often, the patients are old in age.

Kamal: I am a nurse here in this department. It's integral for a successful palliative care team to consist of a doctor, a nurse, and a psychotherapist. We go on many home visits. We see medical patients, many of whom are bedridden, or on feeding tubes, or using urine bags. As much as we attend to the patients, we also make huge efforts with their families. We advise them on how to prepare for and cope with the situation at home. For example, we teach family members how to keep the patient clean—how to clean the mouth, the stool, the urine, et cetera. We tell them about how to prevent and treat bedsores, and how to keep the patient infection-free. Especially in cases where a patient has lung or cheek cancer, hygiene is vital. Hygiene is of utmost importance for anyone who is in the process of dying, actually. We coach on cleaning, keeping everything fresh, and keeping the room clean as well.

Vineeta: Kamal helps with applying the dressing to keep the patient clean. Most of our patients are on some type of tubes, like urine or feeding tubes. Kamal expertly teaches caregivers how to maintain the tubes, empty the urine, and feed the patient. Feeding is actually an art; if the caregiver does not do it properly, it can cause trouble and discomfort to the patient. Kamal also counsels families on the proper diet for patients. Most of our patients are unable to eat—it's a big problem for them, physically and emotionally. They usually don't have much of an appetite, so to present them with options in a careful manner is very important. Prashob actually used to be a chef so he helps too! He speaks to families about how to make the food more interesting, palatable, and good for the patient.

Most of the time, when patients are nearing death they cannot eat much, so we advise them to take everything in the form of drops. The quantity of food is so small, and relatives are always wondering why the patient isn't eating. In Indian culture, love and care is often expressed through food; it also makes families feel a sense of hope when the patient is eating. We have to regularly remind the families that whatever the patient is consuming is what he needs.

The patient's lack of eating is not a rejection of the love being offered by the family. Most patients cannot swallow—that reflex is gone for many. Relatives don't realize it, try to feed their loved one, and the patient chokes. He may feel forced, and the family sometimes feels rejected. Of course, this deeply affects everyone emotionally. When patients stop eating, a sense of impending reality often takes over.

Our work is not just about writing a prescription. It's about seeing the patient as a whole. He's a person who likes to eat, drink, rest, talk, and sleep. He has social needs too—his life isn't, and shouldn't be, just about his pain and suffering.

We are always assisting with the emotional issues of the patients and their families. We deal with many patients who are in the last stages of cancer, or who only have a few more months to live. But we see them as having a span of life left that deserves to be of good quality. How do we achieve that quality of life? By helping the patient emotionally. Anyone who has been diagnosed with a terminal disease may not be at a stage of acceptance. They may have a lot of issues that they aren't even aware of. The fear, the guilt, the shame, worrying about what will happen to their families after their death. They may be scared of pain and how it will feel to die. "Will I choke up? Will it hurt?" This is normal for anyone who's in the last stage of life.

Once we know what they are thinking, we can address their concerns. We also want to always be transparent with the patient. When it is clear they will not survive, their loved ones often tell them, "Things will be fine, just take this medicine," or "We're trying everything we can to save you." The truth is not often revealed to patients by their doctors or caregivers. But we cut through that. We don't give false hope. We don't make them hopeless, either. We show them reality as best we can.

Prashob: Once patients discover that they have an incurable disease, they are at first shocked, or depressed. Our first approach is just to listen to them talk about their feelings. Often, patients will speak about their unfulfilled dreams or their worries, or they'll express their anger and frustration. We try to understand the emotional aspect of a person. It's about being empathetic. Every doctor tries to add days to a patient's life, but we try to add *life* to a patient's *days*. We want the patient to feel, to experience, to be as joyful and blissful as they can be in those days that they have left. Our goal is to help a person live, rather than merely exist.

Vineeta: We know about the process of the body shutting down; relatives and patients do not. Most patients want to know what will happen to them. We use very practical language to explain what the situation is, and to tell them that it could get worse. We tell them about the relief that medications, like patches or suppositories, will provide. We advise the families on how and in what circumstances to administer these medications.

For a person about to die, the most common complaints are pain and problems breathing because their lungs are shutting down. There will be less urine. It may not be possible to swallow food because of dryness of the throat, and sometimes even loss of consciousness. There is pain and swelling all over the body. These are the common symptoms that we explain to the families. We have a number that they can call anytime, even in the night, if they have a question. Patients often call me to ask questions about medications.

Prashob: Emotionally you'll see a difference from person to person. Everyone is suffering—the patient, the family, the friends, the parents—everyone. When we give a patient some drops, it might help to a certain extent, but for a relative, it's a huge relief. "Oh, she's taking five drops, now I can have something to eat."

Psychologically, the family is often more in denial than the patient. The patient, many times, is able to accept his condition, and what is happening to his body. But relatives don't want to accept it. In India, people aren't inclined to talk openly about death. Regularly, we ask the patients' families how they're doing, and almost always, the response is, "*Ekdam theek hain*," or "Everything is totally fine." To accept impending death is very difficult; bringing people into acceptance is a big task. Anticipatory grief starts from the day the patient is diagnosed as palliative. It's just so important to talk about it.

We take care of the patient and his family from the beginning until the end, and even after the patient is gone. We offer bereavement care, or counselling for relatives and family members if they need or want it. When the patient is the sole breadwinner of the household, we offer assistance in financial planning as well.

Death care is so important. We need to psychologically prepare the relatives and the patient, who are at varying levels of acceptance. At the Bhaktivedanta Hospital, we stress the "Five Loving Exchanges" for a patient who is about to die. We find this model to be extremely beneficial, and even miraculous. In order to help a patient pass away peacefully, we encourage families to express these Loving Exchanges:

1. I love you.
2. I know you love me too.
3. Please forgive me for any negative thing I may have done in my life.
4. I forgive you, too.
5. We will remember you always, and never forget you.

We also stress a sixth:

6. We will be okay after you are gone."

There have been so many cases when the patient wouldn't die—it was clear that they were holding on—and then after hearing these Loving Exchanges, the patient was able to pass peacefully. It's so important to clear out the emotional clutter. We carry a lot of baggage with us until the time of death, and we don't always clear it with everyone before we die. During the last or dying stage, people have what we call "death vision." They see their whole life in a rewind form. You can exactly make out from the patient's facial expression what they are going through—they might be smiling, frowning, looking pensive.

If you were in that situation, what would you require? Really think about it—what would you need? You'd need nothing else but a person to show you love, to hold your hand, and to be affectionate and caring. It's not about some therapy or medicine. It's about love and care.

We have patient kits that align with different spiritual beliefs. For practitioners of *bhakti-yoga*, we have some dust from Vrindavan, Ganga water, *tulasi* leaves, *japa* beads, and Mayapur Nrisimhadeva oil.[11] For Muslim patients we have the Quran, *tasbih*, and holy water. For Christians, we have rosaries, and we call a priest. The way patients want to die varies, and we try to accommodate these variations. Again, it's not about artificially administering medicines to expand the life; it's about giving quality of life. We want people to be able to die with dignity. Most people don't really think about this; they think about *living* with dignity, but not really about *dying* with dignity.

In a way, death is glorious for an unalloyed devotee of God, as it's the time he or she will be en route to meet the

---

11. A scented oil offered to the deity of Nrisimhadeva in Mayapur.

Lord. Wouldn't it be nice if we could all die with a smile on our face? Excited to be reunited with God? Srila Prabhupada said that in a way, death for such a devotee is a celebration—a celebration of a person's life, and a celebration of the reunion with God.

Vineeta: Currently, our team consists of the three of us, and a number of volunteers like Ridwan, social workers, and various NGOs. It's mostly the three of us that deal with patients, although we have a lot of support. For example, with Muslim patients, we will often call on our Muslim volunteers to read or pray together with the patient.

I remember one Muslim patient, a man called Farhan. The process of dying took him about four days. Each and every member of the family was with him when he was on his deathbed, including all his children. At all times, one person was reciting prayers and one person was reading the Quran. They read from the chapter that's supposed to be read while someone is dying. The family was so sweet and dedicated; they did this around the clock for four days.

After Farhan passed away, his wife called me and said, "Vineeta, those were the best four days of Farhan's life. Everyone in our family, even our youngest grandchild, was praying and reading for him. Thank you for training us on how to be there for him in that most crucial moment."

Each one of us has been trained in spiritual care. If we have patients in the hospital, the Spiritual Care team takes care of them. We will administer spiritual care to all our home patients ourselves. We also train our volunteers in how to spiritually care for and interact with patients. Most of our volunteers are youngsters, like Ridwan. Death is, of course, very difficult for them—even seeing an open wound can be traumatizing for them. We always accompany them on their first few visits, and once they are comfortable, we allow them to visit patients on their own, with the patient and family's permission.

Patients are just waiting for someone to come and talk to them. Even just for 30 minutes—it really makes their day. If it's appropriate, we try to add something to their day to make it special; sometimes we bring flowers, or balloons, or a small gift. But they really appreciate talking the most. Thankfully, the younger generation absolutely loves talking!

Prashob: Patients really pour their hearts out. They really want someone to come and just listen. They want to talk about their lives. They want to be *asked* about their lives. They want to pass knowledge, especially to the youngsters.

My dad is one of the main reasons I am here. He used to do a lot of social work, even though he was a businessman. Whenever he saw anyone who needed help, he'd be there. Inspired by him, I became a volunteer here in the Palliative Care department. I was working for the Taj Hotel as a chef, and I was content. I had a good salary, and a good work environment. The more I introspected, however, the more I realized that I wanted to do something else with my life. It was actually a patient who made me realize this. He was on his deathbed, and yet he cared enough to ask me, "Is this real happiness you're getting, from the Taj?"

This was the question that changed my life. I started thinking about it. Could I be fulfilled cooking for a restaurant all day? My passion used to be food styling, and I did a lot of it. I thought to myself, "I like this, but is it giving me true happiness?" For me, the answer was no. I was putting a smile on my face every day, but something wasn't right. I realized how happy I felt when I helped a patient through my volunteer work at the Bhaktivedanta Hospital. If I could relieve even one small bit of pain of a dying person, my life would be a success.

So I resigned. Everyone was shocked. My mother disapproved, but my father said he understood and supported me completely.

I went back to school and studied psychology, with an emphasis on counselling so I could obtain the proper qualifications to do it professionally. Now, I am in the process of completing my Masters degree.

Vineeta: Prashob has always been so passionate about helping people. I remember there was one patient that Prashob would visit regularly. Even on his vacation Sundays, he'd tutor the patient's kids. He really got into it, and wanted more patients. He did very well. He would just enter the heart of the patient. Things I wouldn't know as a medical doctor. Prashob would break through all barriers, explore the patient's feelings, and really talk to him and make him feel better.

Prashob: One thing I've noticed is that when patients see that a doctor is coming, they feel nervous and reserved. They know that medicines are not working, and they feel pain. But when they see a friend is coming, someone to listen to them, their mood is completely different. They become eager.

I remember one patient we went to visit. On the first day, he yelled, "Get out! Who called you?" It was his son who had called. "Get out! I don't want any treatment. I'm fine."

"I understand you're going through a lot of pain and problems," I said. "We can give you these medications, if you'd like. They will help you feel better, and then we can come back another time."

"No, don't come back, I never want to see your face again!" he yelled.

The next time we went, he said, "Why are you here?" But his tone was a little softer.

I asked him if he was taking his medication. "No." And that was that.

The third time, he greeted us with, "Oh, you're back again." There was a huge difference in tone. He said he didn't want to take any medicine.

The fourth time we went, he said, in a very gentle tone, "You're not going to leave me, are you?" He added, "What do you want from me?"

"I am here because I really want you to be comfortable and peaceful. I want to hear what's in your heart." And just like that, he poured his heart out. For two hours, he cried and cried, and told me things he said he'd never told anyone before, including his wife and other family members.

I remember another patient who had oral cancer. When he was admitted, there were maggots in his mouth. When I met him, he was crying. Before coming to this hospital, all the doctors who cared for him tried to treat his physical pain. But this man very clearly needed emotional support as well. I spent a lot of time with him, listening to him, and making physical contact. This astonished him; no one was even talking to him, much less touching him. Even his previous doctors, although they all meant well, would feel uncomfortable because maggots would fall on them while they were cleaning him. The doctors would naturally make facial expressions that indicated their shock or disgust with the maggots, and this made the patient feel horrible. The facial expression is so important. As best we can, we have to try to be equipoised; the patient is already in so much pain, and it's our job to help make it better, and to help him cope.

I talked to this man with a smile on my face. Every time I smiled, he smiled. He thanked me profusely. I was so happy for whatever I was able to do for him. That experience really gave me some practical realization that we are not the body—we are the soul that resides inside the body, and our job is to love each other's souls. The body is made of material elements. It's going to disintegrate and decay. So why are we concentrating so much on the body? There was clearly a loving, kind personality inside that body.

The patient went back to his village, where there was a small health centre. An ambulance driver there had compassion for him, and told us that he'd do his dressing for him daily, free of charge. He got supplies from the Bhaktivedanta Hospital and took very good care of the patient until he passed away about two weeks later. The patient had no family; it was the driver who called us to tell us that he passed away. I was grateful to have been able to make him smile.

Vineeta: Many times, patients are alone, with no strong ties with family or friends. Naturally, those patients feel lonely and neglected.

There was one lady named Deepika, who we visited at home. According to her family, she was very controlling. She was a very ambitious, successful executive. In the process of climbing the corporate ladder, she became distant from her husband and children. After some time, her husband left and took the children with him. She didn't fight; she just continued with her successful career.

One day, she was diagnosed with breast cancer. She decided she wouldn't inform anyone—she wanted to continue to manage on her own. She began chemo and radiation therapy, but unfortunately, her cancer only worsened and after a few years, the doctors told her that the treatment was no longer going to help her. Even then, she didn't contact her husband or children. Her neighbours came to her aid, intent on helping her. She told her neighbours that she didn't have the courage to call her family in her condition, because she felt she had wronged them.

"No, they're your family. They'll help you," the neighbours said.

The neighbours contacted Deepika's husband and children, who were then living in England, and told them of her situation. At that point, Deepika's son called me, and told me all about what a controlling woman Deepika was, and how she never wanted to listen to anyone. But he still wanted us to give her care, and to come to India and help.

I met Deepika sometime later in her home. She didn't open up to me. She asked me to just help her manage her pain with medication, which I did. I also answered questions she had about her cancer, and gave her Srila Prabhupada's *Bhagavad-gita As It Is.*

A few days later, I got a call from her son saying that Deepika wanted to come to Bhaktivedanta Hospital based on what I told her about it. I arranged a bed for her. When she arrived, she was amazed by the spiritual atmosphere. The Spiritual Care nurses would talk to her, give her *prasadam*, and read to her. That changed her a lot. She said she was feeling happier, and she even started glowing. The nurses gave her *caranamrita*,[12] and Deepika kept asking for more and more. She stayed for almost a month.

One day, her son called me and told me it was Deepika's birthday. "Can we surprise her?" he asked.

We arranged a small cake and party. People came and chanted Hare Krishna. We sang "Happy Birthday" to her, and she was visibly touched. Her son, daughter, and grandchild were there. We did a cake cutting in her hospital room,

---

12. The liquid mixture used to bathe the deity of Krishna, consisting of milk, ghee (clarified butter), water, and honey.

and she was very thankful. That same night, Deepika asked everyone in her family for their forgiveness.

She said, "Please forgive me, I realize all the pain I put you through. Thank you for helping me at this time. Please accept my apology." The son and daughter hugged her and asked for her forgiveness as well.

Two days later, she left her body. Before she left, she and her husband were speaking to the nurses. Deepika told them, "Please take care of my husband. He's a very nice person. See that he doesn't have any pain. I love him."

And then, she and her husband hugged.

The spiritual ambiance, *prasadam*, and counselling that was given helped changed her heart. She was a very rigid and controlling person, and yet became someone who sincerely asked for forgiveness, while shedding tears.

This story really moved my heart. I thank Krishna for somehow bringing her here. There are so many touching stories here!

Kamal: There was one patient I remember—Beena—who was bedridden in the same room for eight months.

Vineeta: Yes, I remember her. She was feeling very sorry for herself, and was in extreme pain. We put her on morphine.

Prashob: She didn't want to move from her bed, but actually, she was physically capable. As a rule, we avoid extreme sympathy—we don't want to look at the patient and say, "We're feeling so sorry for you and your condition." We want to acknowledge it, acknowledge their feelings and pain, and then help them as best we can.

Vineeta: For this patient, we brought some volunteers, and we stayed with her for hours just to help her get out of her bed. Step by step. "First, sit. Now, move one leg." Every step took almost an hour. But we gave her that time.

Prashob: We had to physically be there to help her; she wouldn't have done it if we just told her to. And she did it! She was so proud of herself! We were all cheering for her. We just took her to the front of her house, and she was so emotional and grateful.

Her condition ran deeper than just not walking. She cried and complained a lot, but it was clear that much of it was to get attention. She thought that if she complained, her son would come and sit next to her. She was not on speaking terms with her daughter-in-law, Shweta. To make things more difficult, they were all living together. Beena didn't exactly make life easy for Shweta. She'd say things like, "This is my room. My kitchen. You can't come in."

Vineeta: One day, I was speaking to Beena and as usual, she started to complain about everything and everyone in her life. "I'm not able to fix all of your problems," I told her. "Why don't you start telling someone who actually may be able to help you?" I gave her a picture of the Radha-Krishna deities in Mayapur. "Whenever you want to talk," I said, "keep this picture in front of you. Radha and Krishna will always be here to help you."

The next time I saw her, she said, "I'm talking to your Radha and Krishna, but I still have so much pain."

"Maybe your cries for God aren't loud enough," I said, honestly. "When a child cries loudly, then surely the parent will pick up the child. Put all your feelings into your crying."

She put the picture of Radha and Krishna in front of her bed. She used to look at it and cry, "Why are you doing this to me? I want to leave this place. Why me?"

Although her conversations with Radha and Krishna were angry, we could see that her heart was starting to soften. Prashob told Beena that he had Radha-Krishna deities at home, and asked if she wanted to make some jewellery for them. She agreed, and started making jewellery for the deities. She also started reading some of Srila Prabhupada's books: *Perfect Questions, Perfect Answers* and *The Laws of Nature*.

Beena was transferred to the Bhaktivedanta Hospital for a few days while her house was being fumigated. While she was at the hospital, something changed. "Why are you wearing *tilak*? I want some too. Why are you Hare Krishnas all wearing neck beads?[13] Can I wear them as well?" She didn't want to leave.

Prashob: When Beena was staying here at the hospital, she told us she was truly happy. She loved it here so much. Her son asked if he could volunteer here because he saw the positive effect the hospital was having on his mother. Beena even started praying to Krishna for the happiness of her daughter-in-law. She went from being abusive to becoming busy with chanting, making jewellery for the deity, and telling her friends all about her Krishna. We were able to take her to the temple across the road, which she enjoyed thoroughly.

She went back home, and her pain became manageable. She and Shweta started to be more civil towards each other. For example, Beena finally let Shweta cook for her. They even invited us all over for dinner one day.

After some time, Beena's condition deteriorated. We went for a visit, and discovered that she would likely pass away within the week. We put on some chanting in the background. Beena started to smile, and said, "Krishna, Krishna." We said to her, "We're here, don't worry."

We put *tilak* on her forehead and made sure she was wear-

---

13. Many Hare Krishna devotees wear neck beads made from the *tulasi* (holy basil) plant, as a form of protection.

ing her *tulasi* neck beads. We kept the chanting speakers close to her ears. She was very peaceful.

Before she passed away, I encouraged her to have a heart-to-heart with Shweta to clear up the tension between them. Beena had only hugged Shweta once, on her wedding day. I said, "As you open your heart towards her, she will open her heart towards you as well." At first, Beena said, "No, this is not possible."

"There's not a lot of time left," I said soberly.

Two days before Beena passed away, she and Shweta cried in each other's arms, and forgave each other for any misgivings.

Beena really understood that her pain belonged to her body, and that her soul was actually blissful. She was so tuned into the chanting—it was plain to see. She kept saying "Krishna, Krishna."

Vineeta: When I think about the person she was when we first visited, and the person she became, it's remarkable. She was totally changed.

Her son told us he was so thankful, as he didn't imagine that his mother would be peaceful and emotionally pain-free at the time of death. He said she looked like an angel when she passed.

"Thank you for giving me my mother back," he said.

This is what palliative care is. We are always trying to learn more about care, communication, and compassion. We are always practicing love and acceptance.

When I look back on my privilege of serving patients here, I feel so thankful to Srila Prabhupada.

Prashob: When you feel like you've achieved the goal of your life, like this is the service you were meant to do, grab it, do it, and don't look back. It's the most fulfilling and amazing feeling in the world.

Journal Entry: With the Palliative Care Team

Radha Bhakti
January 23, 2014

I am just finishing up my lunch with the inspiring Palliative Care team and we are about to leave when an elderly gentleman enters the canteen and sits at the table next to us. His eyes are warm and loving, and everyone at the table, including me, greets him with smiles and "Hare Krishna."

He looks at me and says, "I haven't seen you before—are you new here?"

"Yes, *Prabhu*, I'm just here for a volunteer project," I say with a smile. "How about you? Do you work here?"

"No," he says. "But I've been involved with this project since the beginning. I used to have get-togethers at my home. The founding doctors used to come. At that time, they weren't interested in philosophy. All they wanted was *prasadam!*"

We all laugh. Something about this man is so charming.

"You know, I am 77 years old," he says. "My wife passed away here just a few months ago. I just wanted to come here for lunch."

He came here for lunch? I think. *His wife passed away here and he came here for lunch?*

"I'm so sorry to hear about your wife," I say. "I can't imagine what you're going through. How are you doing, *Prabhu?* Are you alright?"

"*Dekho*,"[14] he says solemnly. "There is a picture of my wife hanging on the wall at home. I don't look at it."

A rush of compassion comes over me. What is it about this man that makes me feel like I can talk to him for hours?

---

14. The meaning of *dekho* is "you see."

"It must be difficult for you to be here," I say.

"I like coming here," he says. "It's peaceful. And I like meeting the various people here and talking to them. And today, Krishna sent me you to talk to!"

Likely sensing that I don't want to leave, Vineeta says, "I'm sorry, *Prabhu*, we should get going. We are just about to go for some home visits."

"Yes, of course, please go," the man says, smiling.

As we are collecting our belongings and getting ready to leave, I say, "What is your name, *Prabhu?*"

He reaches into his wallet and hands me his card. "My name is Mahaprabhu Das," he says, with folded palms to offer respect. "Let's meet again, so we can speak some more."

"Of course," I say, also folding my palms. "Hare Krishna."

We may have spoken for five minutes, but this man completely captured my heart.

⚘

I didn't know what to expect when we visited a number of palliative patients in their homes today, but I didn't expect it to be joyful. I felt *joyful*. What a difference it makes to patients and their families when this team visits them! Patients were smiling, laughing, talking. It was clear that this was the highlight of their day. The energy Ridwan brought was amazing. While the rest of us were listening to the patients and their families speak about symptoms and feelings, Ridwan was making them smile by being his youthful and entertaining self. To one 90-something year old patient, he just said, "Auntie! Selfie!" and put his arm around her and clicked away. And I watched this elderly woman, who didn't even know what a selfie was, become completely endeared by the charm of this dynamic young man and the silliness of a selfie. Her face lit up, and she laughed unexpectedly and heartily.

It wasn't easy for me to be around so many sick people, to witness their pain, and to hear about the sorrows of the ones they will leave behind. It wasn't easy for me to be brought into people's grief-stricken worlds, with all the accompanying sights and smells. And yet, I didn't want to leave.

We visited six patients and their families. Somehow, after all of this, I feel more connected to God than I ever have. Somehow, I feel that this is the most valuable service to him—to provide love and affection to his children, especially those who are about to leave their bodies.

When I go to Bandra on the weekend, I will speak to my family about making the arrangements for my uncle, on his deathbed, a little different, a little more devotional. Somehow now, I understand more of what he's going through.

While the Palliative Care team gave so much to everyone they met today, their own hearts, and mine, were completely full by the end of the day.

Interview with Dr. Ashok Shetty

Dermatologist and Medical Coordinator
January 24, 2014

The Beginnings

I met all the founding doctors in the late '80s at the Chowpatty temple. By that time, I had already completed my post-graduate degree in Dermatology. I remember meeting Dr. Vivek Shanbhag at the temple, and being instantly drawn to his positivity and optimism, and I wanted some of that. So, I befriended him. He was wonderful, always patiently answering my questions. In those days, I wasn't really interested in spirituality, but I would occasionally go to the temple with my wife who was much more spiritual than I was. I was really inspired by the level of her faith.

Because I am a doctor, Vivek and the other doctors would ask me to join them at their camps. I was already a practicing dermatologist and I had a young son at home, so typically I'd go with them only on Sundays when I could spare some time. I went most often to the camp in Palghar. Slowly, my connection to this project and to all the doctors grew.

The hospital was built much later, in 1998. I was still associated with the project and assisting the doctors on weekends. After the hospital was built, I thought I'd come once or twice a week to lend my services, outside of my regular dermatology practice. I was living about 30 km south of here. In Mumbai, travelling 30 km takes much longer than it might in another city—everything here takes at least three times as long. It was hard for me to come here more than once or twice a week. As time passed, though, I found myself coming more and more. Whether it was to consult for a patient, or to hear a class from Radhanath Swami who was coming often, there was always a reason to come back. Soon it was twice, then three times a week. It wasn't my plan; it just started happening. To spend my days working in the field that I love, while simultaneously feeling spiritually nourished, and having the opportunity to pass that spirituality to others, was a very special and divine experience. I felt a sense of fulfilment that I hadn't before.

In the early 2000s, Dr. Sankhe asked me if I'd be interested in taking up a management role. I was very reluctant, as I didn't feel qualified. But I also wanted to serve. I told Dr. Sankhe that I would do it if he couldn't find anyone else.

A month later, he was still asking me to consider taking the position of Medical Coordinator. Reluctantly, and with no experience, I said yes. I had no idea what my job was. Dr. Sankhe told me that I just needed to ensure that patients and doctors are happy. To this day, that is still how I describe my job!

※ ※ ※ ※

A Culture of Care

Patients are the most important people to walk through our doors. My job is to ensure that they are getting proper treatment, and that they are happy with the service we provide. In the beginning, I was working alone but now I have a team of people who help me speak to patients.

Around the world, patient satisfaction is becoming increasingly important. Patients are more empowered than ever before with greater access to medical information and opinions. Doctors are the primary representatives of our hospital to patients, so we are constantly monitoring how satisfied patients are with their doctors and nurses.

We take patient satisfaction very seriously, and we also want to ensure that the staff is happy. Housekeeping staff, doctors, nurses, administrative staff, everyone. Are we providing nice food for everyone? Is it clean? Are they satisfied professionally and personally by working here?

Due to the nature of my role, people will talk to me about the ways they are happy, and the areas they see for improvement. I consider myself very fortunate to have this service. I basically do whatever I can to ensure our staff is peaceful, using their skills nicely, and therefore giving the best results to every patient.

I assist also in the interviewing and selection of consultants. Consultants are most often medical professionals that have a specialty that we lack here at the hospital. For example, a neurosurgeon may come from abroad for his or her own professional development and personal satisfaction. In Peter Burwash's book "Key to Leadership," he says that if he hires a person, he looks for a person with an American's enthusiasm, a Japanese person's attention to detail, and a Thai person's warmth. He's a big inspiration for me.

At one time, there was a world-famous pediatric surgeon who used to practice in the same area as my dermatology practice many years ago. He started coming here to Bhaktivedanta Hospital regularly, because he said it used to provide him with peace. How wonderful, and bizarre at the same time, when you think about it! He travelled very far, just to sit in the halls of this hospital, because he found it to be peaceful. He also started to volunteer his services. This man drives a fancy car and is affiliated with the most eminent hospitals in the world, but would still volunteer his services here.

Everyone in the material world is suffering—even this famous, affluent doctor. To be able to provide a peaceful environment amidst the chaos is very significant. And that this peaceful environment is found in a hospital is even more special.

At the same time, it's a big challenge to run a hospital. Every day, there are miracles that happen here, and every day there are challenges. The body is always acting in unexpected ways. Sometimes a patient deteriorates unexpectedly, and relatives react in different ways—people go through so many emotions. Once, a staff member's father-in-law came in, complaining of some nausea. Within two days, he was put on a ventilator due to some complications found on the ECG. He walked in and he never walked out.

That loss was particularly hard for me, because the patient's daughter-in-law was a staff member who had so much faith in me. I felt like we disappointed her. It was difficult, but it was an important lesson in Krishna consciousness—I am simply not the controller. I can't take credit for a patient's recovery any more than I can blame myself for a patient's death, as long as I'm genuinely working hard and trying my best. You never know what can happen. Being a doctor, I realize every day that I am merely an instrument.

My job is to do my absolute best to provide the best medical care possible, and in a loving way. Radhanath Swami says that at all levels there should be compassion. He says that compassion, medical efficiency, cleanliness, and good management have to be prominent. He says that we should never forget the purpose for which this hospital was built—to provide true holistic care. That means to tend to the physical, mental, social, and spiritual needs of each patient.

My Vision

It's my aspiration that in the future, we will be known as one of the best hospitals in the world. Not because we have the best technology, but because we have the most caring staff. In my view, we will be the shining example of care based on compassion and love, versus profits and prestige. When patients are receiving various opinions from different doctors, we will be the hospital they trust the most, to receive the advice that is truly in their best interest. We will be the most trusted hospital in the world. People will not be misled; they will have so much faith in us.

This is possible. All we have to do is continuously strive to be pure in heart. This is why we came to Krishna consciousness, isn't it? To become pure in heart. So we have to actually achieve that, with no other motivation than to help others. This compassion should be everywhere—in the nurses, the attendants, security staff, billing folks—everyone should be caring and loving.

We have been given so much by Radhanath Swami and Srila Prabhupada. Srila Prabhupada exemplified compassion and care in his own life—and this is the definition of hospitality—compassion and care.

This is our mission: With love and devotion, we will offer everyone modern scientific holistic care.

We want to transform hearts. After patients come here, they should never be the same again. When a patient goes home, he should be a better person—one with more compassion, patience, self-awareness, and love.

To the degree that we can attain this purity, we are successful.

Another of our missions is to conquer death, at least in a manner of speaking. In our hospital, we have about 7-8 deaths a month, all in the ICU. Of course, every time there is a death, there is a death audit. To conquer death does not mean to prevent it from happening. To conquer death, means to become fearless of death. People come into any hospital out of a fear of death, even if it's just a health checkup. If we can help people to understand that death is part of their spiritual journey, and that it can be glorious, then we consider ourselves successful. We want to help people live their lives in meaningful ways, so that at the time of death they can be peaceful and fearless.

The first lesson in *bhakti-yoga* philosophy is that we are not these bodies, but we are the souls inside these bodies. The soul has a very loving relationship with God. Many doctors need scientific evidence of these things, naturally, as they are trained in science and often feel that religion and spirituality are not credible. But actually, there is so much empiric and scientific evidence that the soul is different from the body. Out-of-body experiences are just one example. It's my dream that we can have a Thanatology department, which means the study of death. This department will be the global leader in scientific research, documenting out-of-body and near-death experiences. We have already started the research process, to document and verify out-of-body experiences and memories from previous lives. In the U. S., there are many journals about near-death experiences. We can contribute, or have our own journals, offering the *bhakti-yoga* perspective. We have the knowledge; we just have to share it with the world.

One day I'd love if we could offer even the most specialized and sophisticated healthcare for free, including heart surgeries and chemo. Can you imagine how pleased

Prabhupada would be? I dream that one day we will receive enough donations to treat the poor for free, regardless of what their condition is, and how specialized their required care is. My dream is that rich patients feel inspired to pay the market rate for the services they receive, thus allowing us to treat those who can't pay without any charge. Everyone, regardless of socio-economic status, will want to be treated here because we will always have the best, most caring doctors.

My dream is also that the most qualified doctors in the world will come for some time and work for free. There are so many doctors around the world who would be willing to do it for their own professional development and satisfaction. We've had some of that already—doctors from America come for a week and work for no charge. The dream is to get the best doctors, generate enough income, and attract donations from well-wishers.

I think this is Radhanath Swami's desire, and I'm sure it will happen. It's just a matter of time! And I hope I'm around to see it!

There are so many advancements in medical technology and hospital management all the time. I don't know if we can always keep up. But if we have the heart, attitude, care, and compassion, this will be the real glory of Bhaktivedanta Hospital.

If we receive people well, then transformations of heart can continue to occur. Radhanath Swami says that the spiritual component to healthcare is the "1" in front of so many zeroes—this is the component of healthcare that gives all other types of care meaning.

I'm very grateful to Srila Prabhupada; it's because of him that we are here today. I am from Udupi and you are from Toronto, but we are sitting here on Mira Road together talking about spirituality and holistic care. This is our great fortune. This is not an activity of this world—we need each other's help and association. Let's wish each other the best, and keep inspiring each other by talking about our dreams for serving Krishna by helping people!

Interview with Dr. Komal Dalal

Doctor and Spiritual Care Leader
February 6, 2014

I met the founding doctors in 1990, about a year after I became a Hare Krishna devotee. My initial focus when joining the hospital was on Spiritual Care and acupuncture. In 2012, however, we realized that there was a dire need for a research department. Since then, I've been leading a team in conducting research and publishing our results. At the moment, we are conducting research on the effects of spiritual care in cancer patients, and on patients suffering from anxiety and depression. So far, our results have been promising.

I'm so motivated when I see the way people's lives change by coming in contact with this hospital. Especially through the Spiritual Care nurses, patients receive so much love and affection, and it really has far-reaching effects, physically, emotionally, and mentally.

❧ ❧ ❧ ❧

Patient Stories

I'm remembering Jayapataka Swami, a renowned Hare Krishna monk, who has been a patient here. When I first started treating him, he was in very bad shape—he had no sensation in his body after having been unconscious for two and a half months as a result of a stroke. I was treating him with acupuncture, and as a result, he immediately felt 25% sensation in his body. Even in his condition, he was so enthusiastic, hopeful, and dedicated to sharing *bhakti* with people around the world. It was very emotional for me to see.

He always asked us to tell him patient stories—stories of lives that changed as a result of coming in contact with Bhaktivedanta Hospital. I started telling him stories about patients while giving him treatment, and it really enlivened him.

While Jayapataka Swami was very ill, Radhanath Swami called him to show his love and support. Almost as a formality, as a way of showing Jayapataka Swami how loved he is, Radhanath Swami invited him to Pune to attend a big festival. It wasn't possible—he was bedridden and practically paralyzed.

But Jayapataka Swami took the invitation seriously—he was determined and insistent. We were panicking. There were way too many risks, and we didn't want Jayapataka Swami to go. We had no idea how to honour what these great personalities wanted and at the same time look after Jayapataka Swami's health!

We called in one of the most senior physicians in Mumbai, a Doctor Tilve. We were sure he would convince Jayapataka Swami that he shouldn't go. But after his meeting with the Swami, Dr. Tilve said to us, "This person's very life and soul is caring for others by sharing *bhakti*. His blood pressure is fluctuating a lot—but I really feel that if you give him what he wants, it will become stable. This is his very purpose."

We were shocked. Against all better judgement, we took Jayapataka Swami to Pune. And he was so excited. Still, he was almost completely paralyzed. It was so difficult to see him like that. He was completely dependent on so many people. To raise a hand, to get out of bed, to eat. Most people would become depressed in this condition, and not want to go anywhere. But not him. He was so enthusiastic. He couldn't even speak; we had a speech therapist from Spain helping him to speak again. In the beginning, whatever he said was a little difficult to understand. But he kept going. I remember being in awe of his humility and enthusiasm. It touches my heart very deeply. On that trip, Jayapataka Swami, with an interpreter, spoke to a crowd of thousands for over two hours from a stretcher. He had the whole crowd in tears because of his love and devotion. His entire life is dedicated to caring for others, even in the compromised state he was in at the time. I'll never forget that. He just embodies care for others.

Another personality that really affected me was Mahavishnu Swami. One evening I received a call that he was in the hospital with severe pain, and that he required acupuncture. He was here for a lung infection, and other illnesses due to his advanced age. He was here for quite some time, and his disciples from all over the world came to meet him. As his condition became more complex, it became clear that he didn't have much time left. He went to Nasik, as he felt that was where he wanted to die. It is the place where he was raised, and where Lord Rama performed many of his pastimes. After he left, however, we got a call that actually he wanted to come back here to Bhaktivedanta Hospital. He said this is just like a holy place and he wanted to leave his body here. I had the opportunity to serve him again as his acupuncturist. Every day, he was surrounded by so many devotees, but on the actual day he left his body, only Dr. Sankhe and I were here. Even the majority of the founding doctors weren't here that day. We had the bittersweet service of applying the *ganga jal*[1], *tulasi*, and *vraja raj* on his body, and we also put a *tulasi* plant next to him. And then, he left us peacefully. It was a profound experience for me.

There was another patient called Kirtida who really

---

1. Sacred water from the river Ganga; it is considered to be very auspicious to have a drop of this water on the tongue at the time of leaving one's body.

inspired me. She was a very senior devotee at the Radha-Gopinath Temple as a counsellor. She was diagnosed with breast cancer three years ago. She underwent surgery, chemotherapy, and radiation, but still, the cancer wouldn't be beat. She was admitted in Bhaktivedanta Hospital as a palliative care patient. She was always smiling, and she kept saying she was ready to die. At one point, there was no other treatment we could give her, so her family took her home for her final days. There was a very spiritual atmosphere there. One day towards the end of January, she began to feel a little breathless and she told her family, "I think I am leaving my body now; give me my clicker."[2] They put *ganga jal* and *tulasi* on her, she was chanting Hare Krishna, and she left. Just like that, sitting on a chair. The previous day, Radhanath Swami went to meet her and he spoke to her for 45 minutes. She used to translate the Swami's classes in Hindi for many devotees. She was at peace and completely lucid, chanting Hare Krishna, when she left. This is such a rare, and fortunate way to leave the body.

✤ ✤ ✤ ✤

Future Vision

These patients and so many more continue to demonstrate that spiritual care makes such a huge difference, especially at the time of death. My vision for the hospital is for it to become famous for spiritual care in particular. Other hospitals should come here and learn the methodology and pay it forward. If we can share this model with many more doctors and nurses around the world, it would

---

2. A device *bhakti-yoga* practitioners use to count the number of times they chant the Hare Krishna *maha-mantra*, when they don't have their prayer beads.

have far-reaching effects. Patients want to listen to their doctors. Especially when the doctors themselves are grounded, compassionate, happy, and healthy people. The spiritual care model here is so effective—I want it to be known everywhere. My dream is that the Bhaktivedanta Hospital name is known in all medical journals around the world. I'm not saying this because I want to be famous—I'm saying this because I think Srila Prabhupada should be famous. All we are doing here is implementing his vision, his philosophy—to bring spirituality to the masses to make for a more peaceful world. Materially, we all have different designations—male, female, doctor, lawyer, Hindu, Christian, Indian, American—but spiritually, we are all the same.

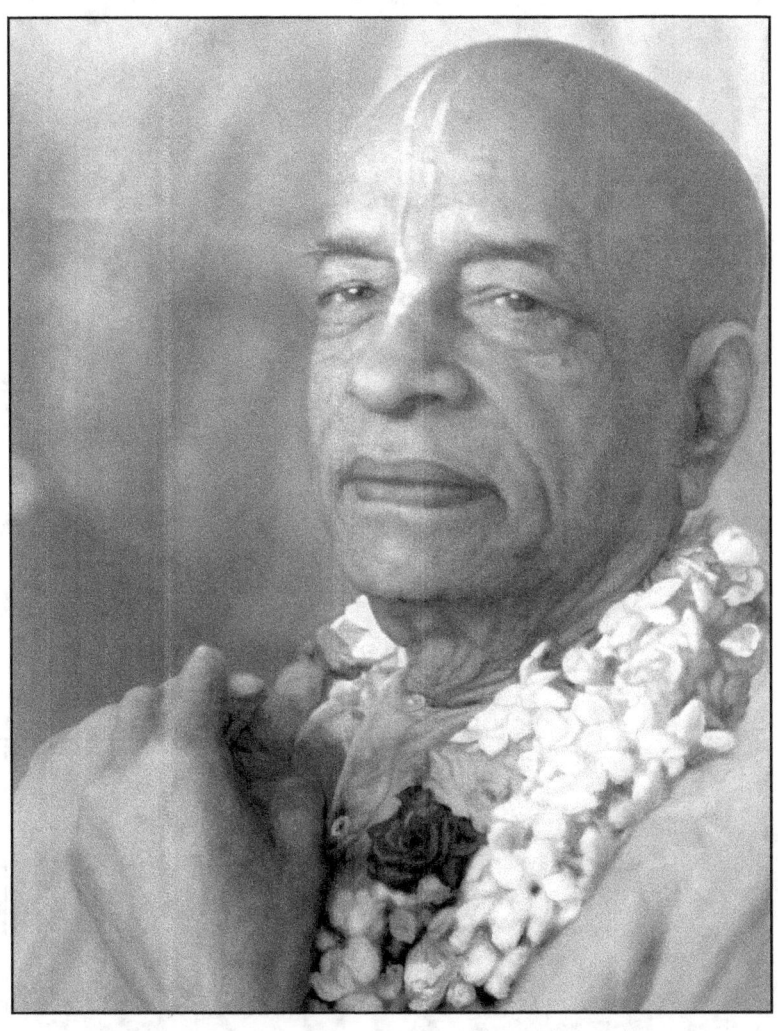

A.C. Bhaktivedanta Swami Prabhupada
He brought *bhakti* outside of India to the rest of the world, and is the Founder-*Acharya* of the International Society for Krishna Consciousness. He is the inspiration behind Bhaktivedanta Hospital.

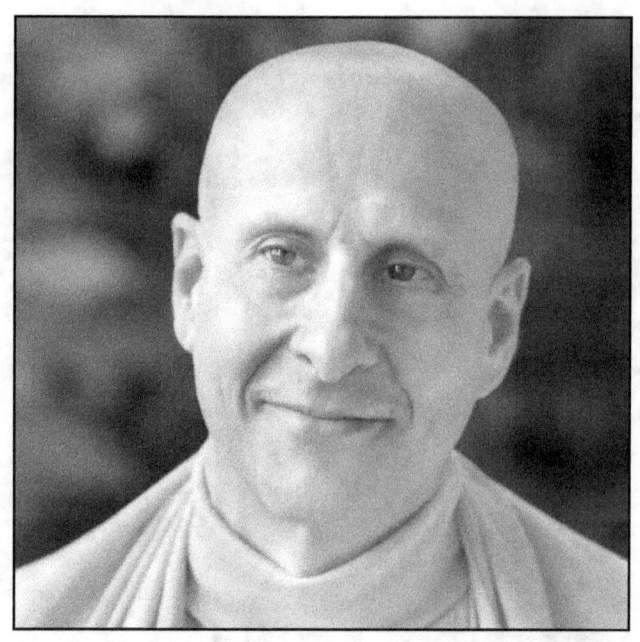

Radhanath Swami is a disciple of Srila Prabhupada, and the spiritual guide of the founding doctors of Bhaktivedanta Hospital.

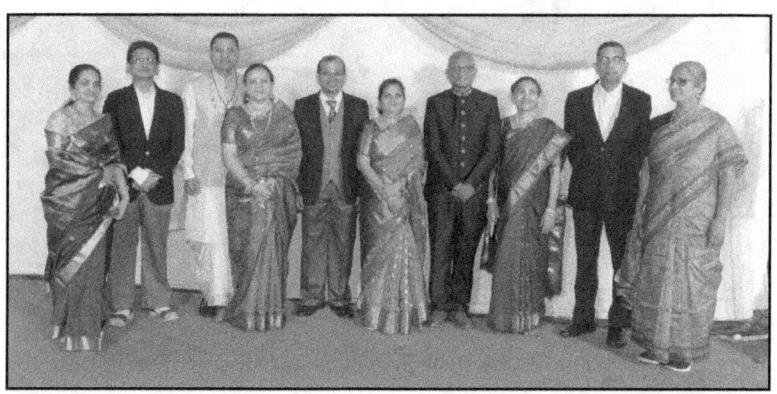

Attending the 25th Anniversary of Bhaktivedanta Hospital in 2023 are (from left): Dr. Kshama Shah, Dr. Bimal Shah, Dr. Vivek Shanbagh, Archana Shanbagh, Dr. Dhaval Dalal, Vaishali Dalal, Dr. Girish Rathod, Smita Rathod, Dr Ajay Sankhe, and Dr. Urmila Sankhe.

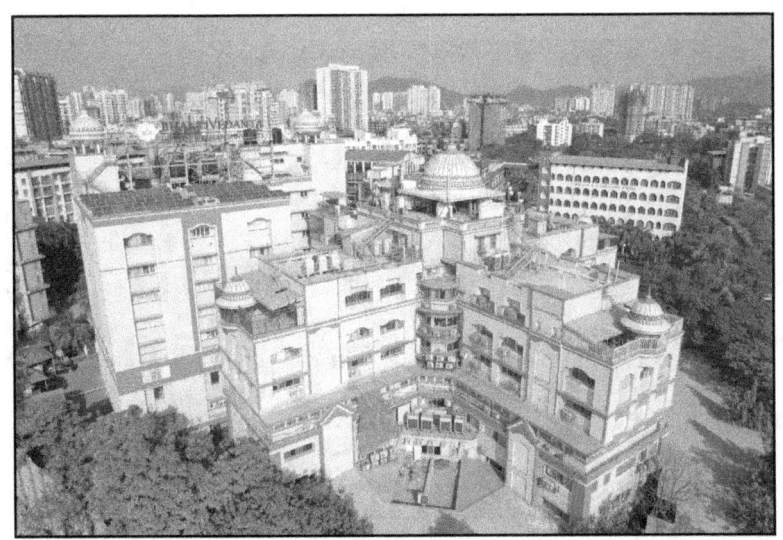

Drone photo of the Bhaktivedanta Hospital in Mumbai, India.

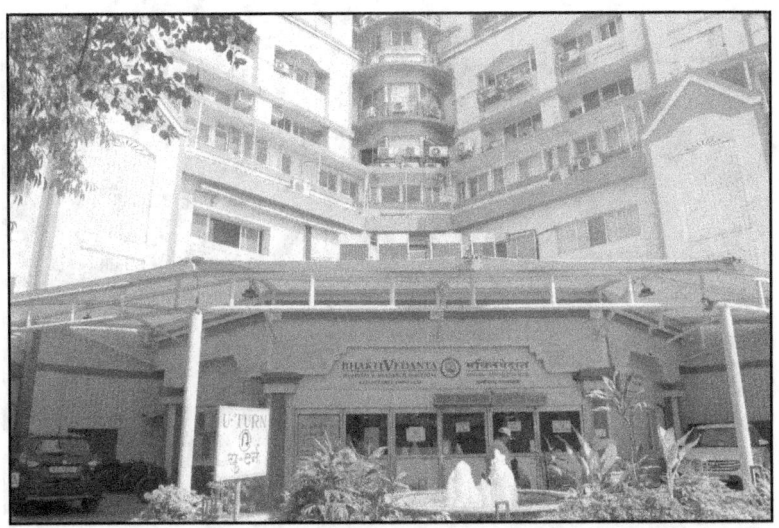

Front entrance to the Hospital

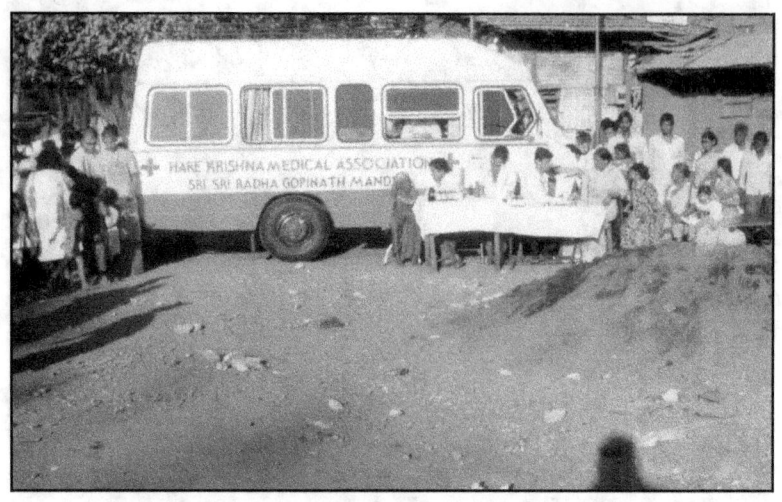

Pictured is one of the first camps that provided medical care to outlying villages.

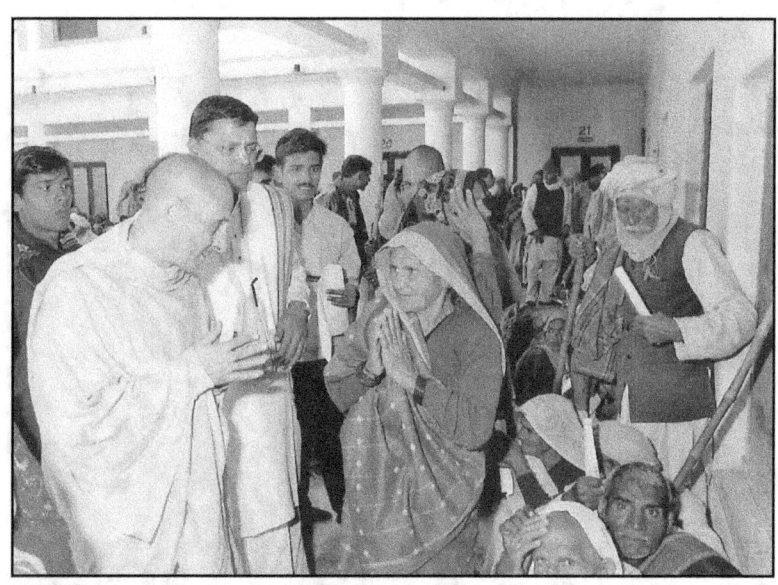

Radhanath Swami visits Barsana eye camps in the early 2000s. Dr. Vivek Shanbagh is standing to the Swami's left.

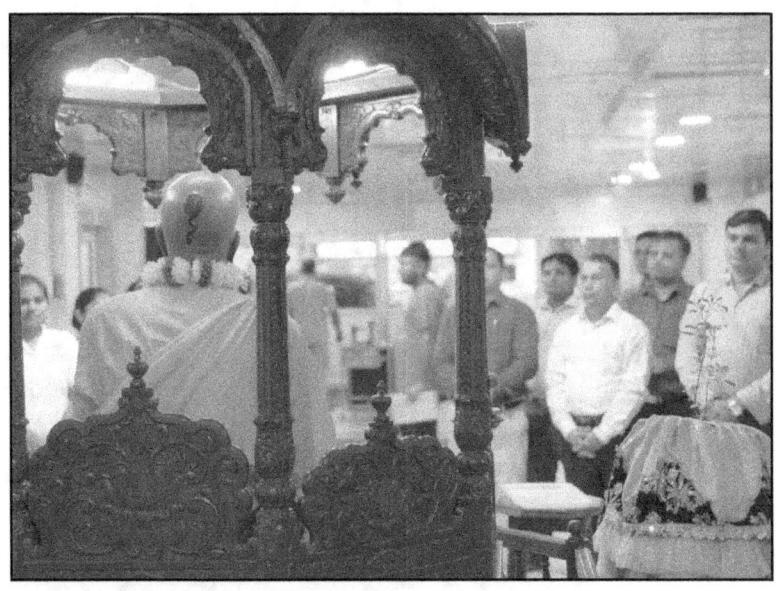

Hospital staff gathers multiple times each day in the main lobby before the deity of Srila Prabhupada for prayers.

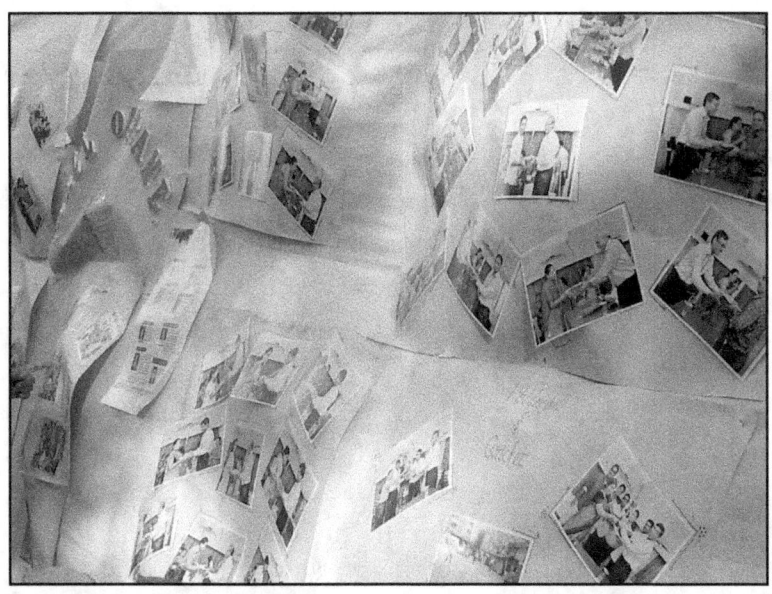

The wall of appreciation at the 2014 Annual Day.

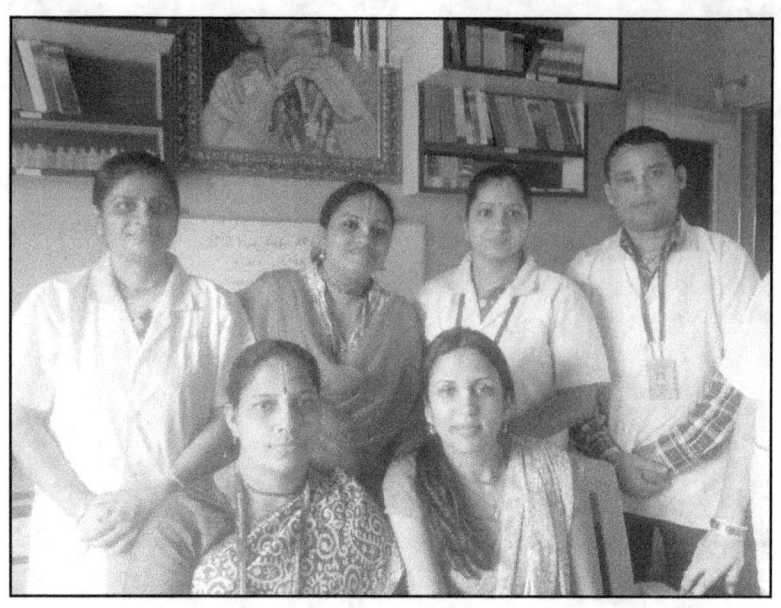

The author with members of the Spiritual Care Team.

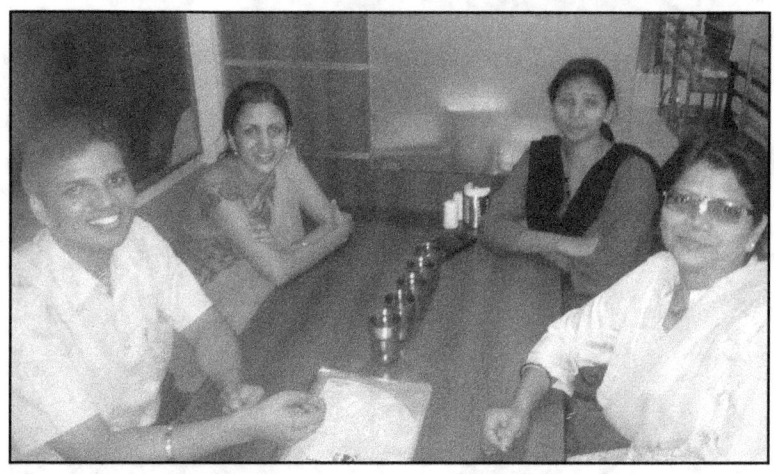

The author talks with the Palliative Care Team.
L-R: Prashob, Radha Bhakti, Kamal, and Vineeta.

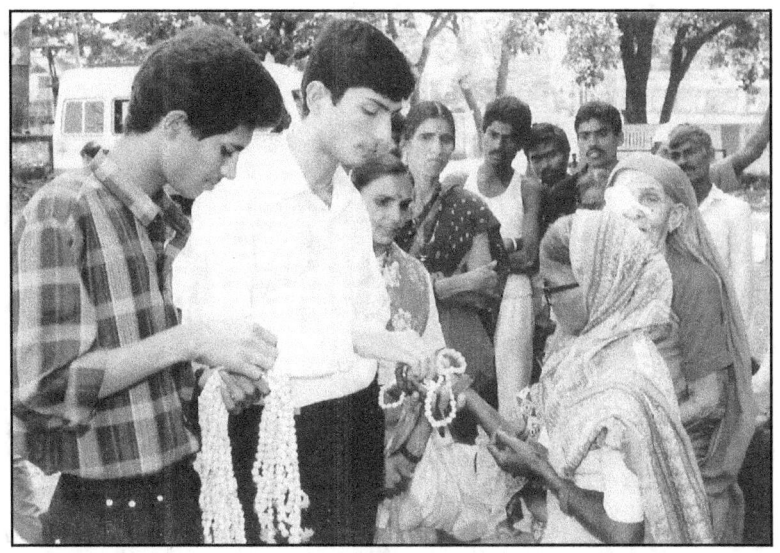

Administering a free mobile clinic, Dr. Ajay Sankhe is second from the left. Circa early-mid 1990s.

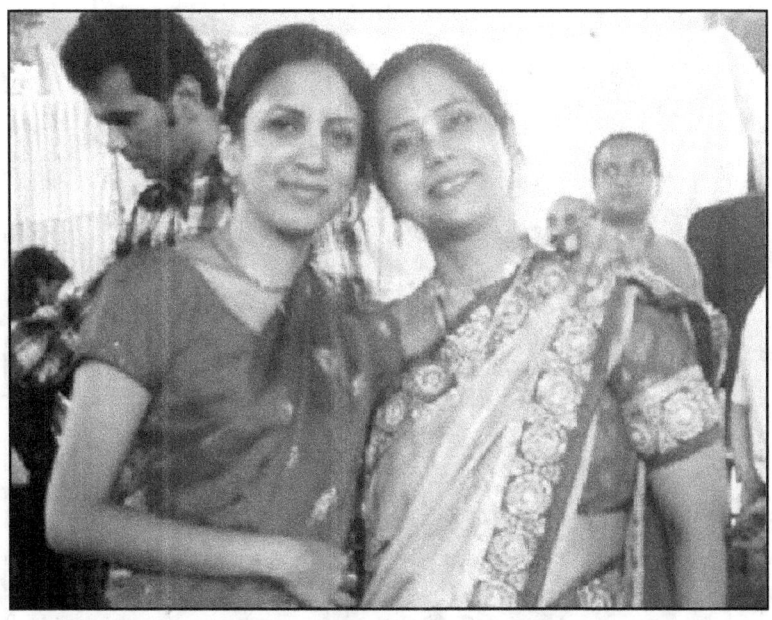

The suthor (left) is with Dr. Komal Dalal, at the wedding of Dr. Vivek Shanbagh's daughter.

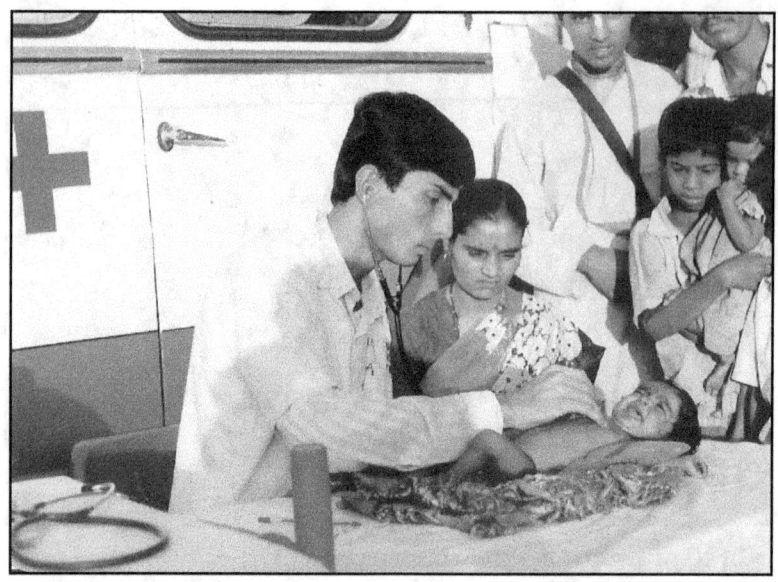

Dr. Sankhe performing an examination at a free mobile clinic, with an ambulance if needed.

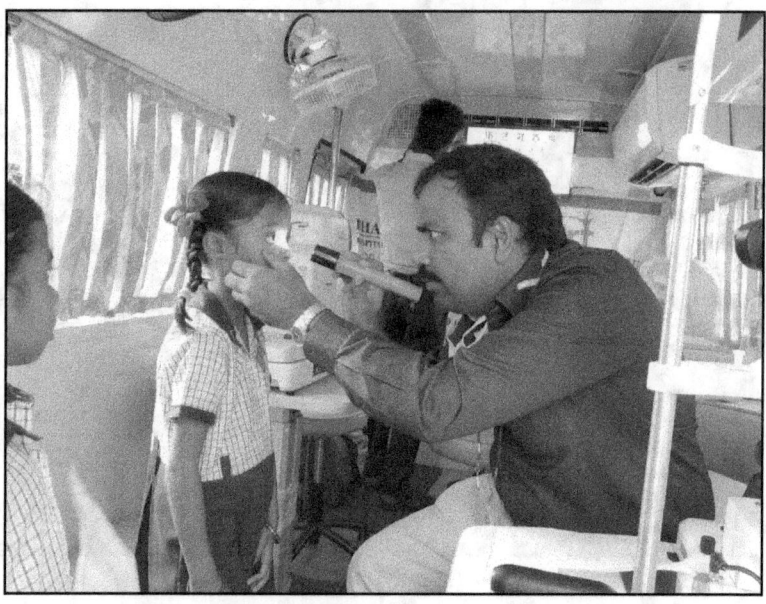

Examinations are given at school children camps.

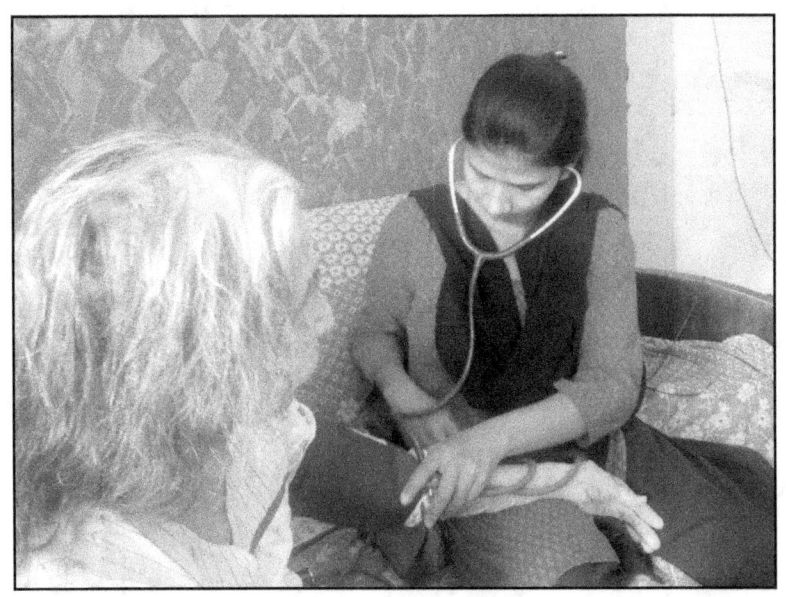

Kamal from the Palliative Care Team checks a patient.

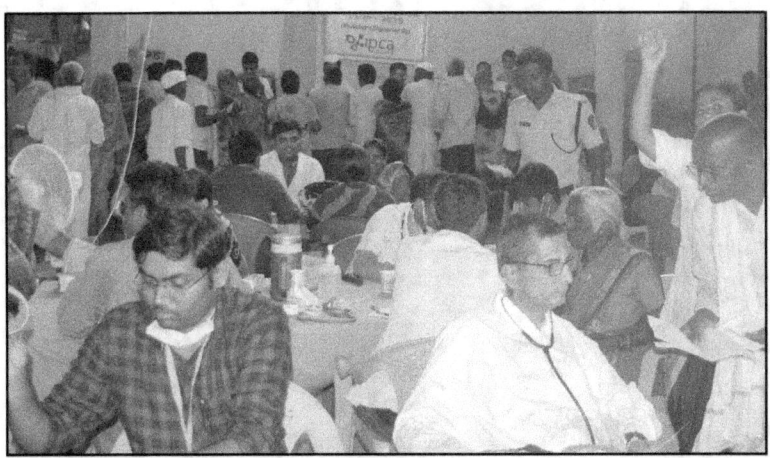

Dr. Sankhe examining patients at a crowded Pandharpur camp.

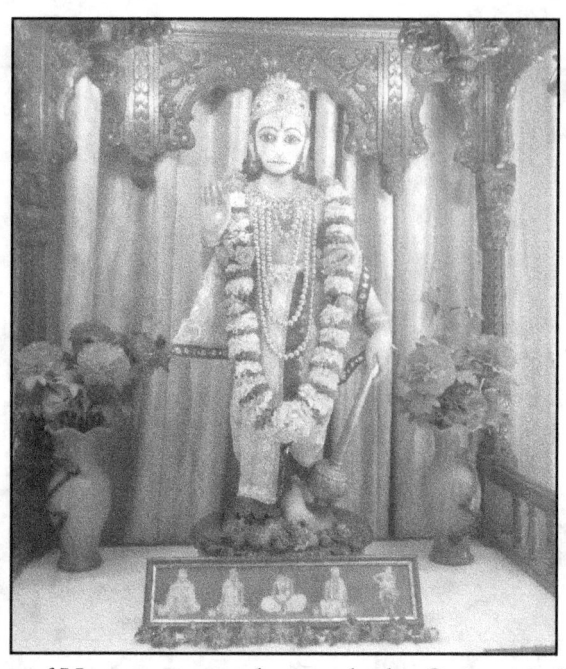

The deity of Hanuman stands outside the Operation Theatre.

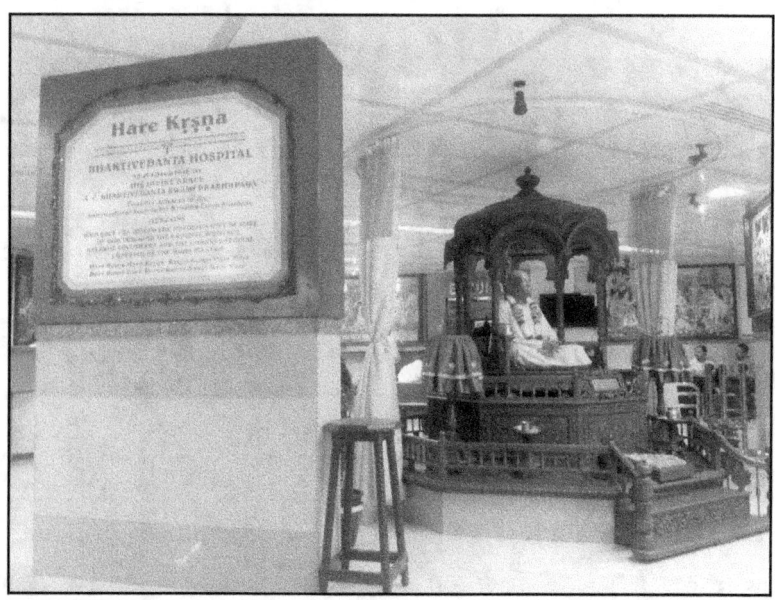

The deity of Srila Prabhupada is in the main lobby.

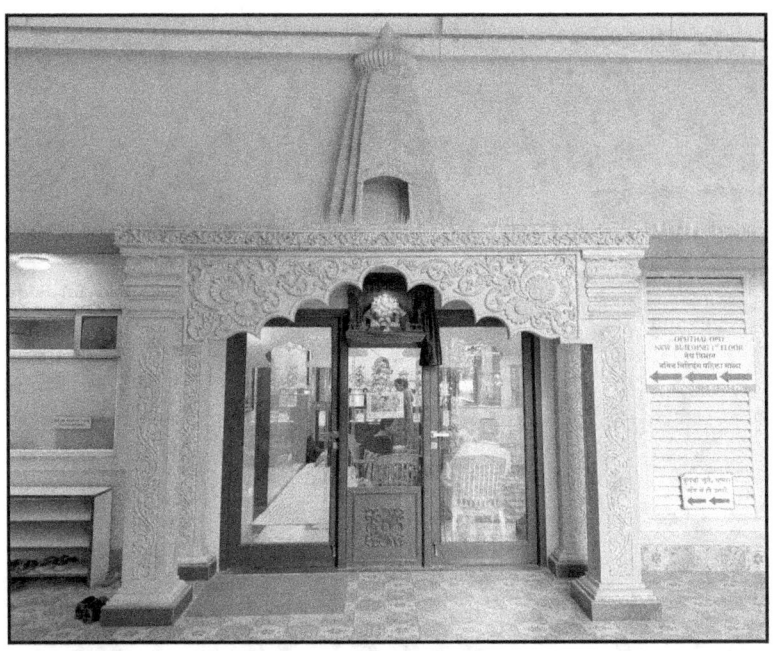

The hospital temple entrance invites people in to worship.

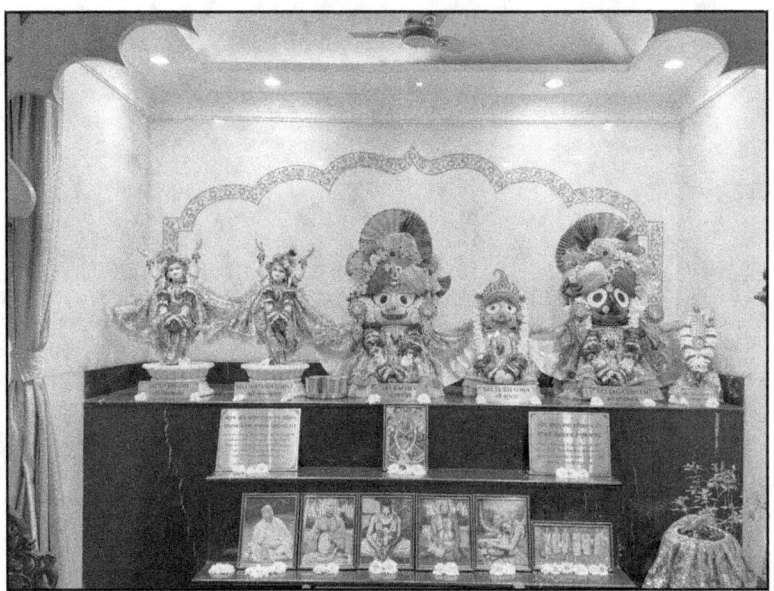

The temple altar is always beautiful.

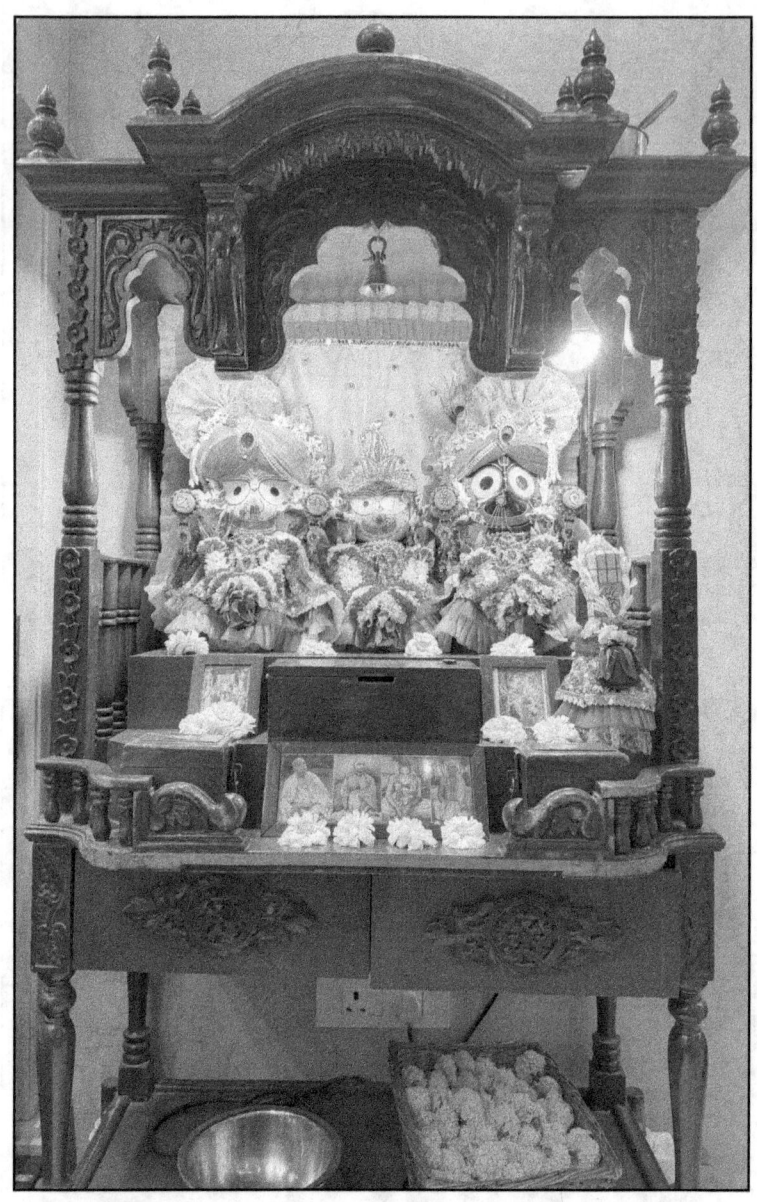

The rolling cart housing the deities of Jagannath (right), Baladeva (left), and Subhadra (middle). This cart is rolled into patient rooms every day for those who want to offer flowers.

Interview with Rakesh and Neha Chopra

Former patients
January 16, 2014

Rakesh: I was born in Allahabad into a large family; I am one of six children—four boys and two girls. In our village, people used to think that having a daughter was a burden, due to having to give a dowry at the time of marriage. Neha and I got married when we were around 15 or 16 years old. At that time in our village, it was considered ideal to do the *kanya-daan*[1] ceremony before a girl began her menstrual cycle. Today, it's not like that. But in those days, a girl would be promised to a boy by the age of 10 or 11. She wouldn't even know what marriage was. She would move in with the boy and his family a few years later. Our parents paired us together because we both came from *brahmana* families.

Neha: In our time, it didn't matter if we didn't like our spouse. It wasn't that you could test out the marriage and then give up after a couple of months if you didn't like it. You had to spend your life with that person. We are happy now, but it took us a while to get to this place.

Rakesh: I'm not sure how long we've been married. Maybe 40 or 41 years. Maybe more. I am 57 years old, I think. In the village, there was no hospital. Even my parents don't know my birthday. They say things like, "You were born on the day that it rained really hard." It might have been in May or June. In our day, no one read horoscopes for the child or anything. A priest would come to the home and bless the child, and the parents would give some charity in honour of their newborn child.

---

1. A ceremony that includes giving away a bride to a groom's family.

We were quite poor growing up. Our parents sent the boys to school, but there was no real emphasis on education; we went to school whenever we felt like it, but the priority was to find work and help support the family. For example, if it were raining too hard, our parents would tell us not to go.

Neha: Us girls weren't even allowed to leave the house. I never went to school. I was raised to learn how to run a house, and then get married.

Rakesh: Although I went to school, I never learned how to read. I didn't go very regularly; there was always something in the house to do. Plus, it was very expensive to go to school.

We now have two sons, aged 26 and 18. One day in 2008, our younger son fell ill. He had very serious jaundice, at the age of 12. He was vomiting a lot. One night he vomited in his sleep, and it produced a vile stench. We weren't sure what was wrong, so we took him to a hospital in Borivali. The doctor told us to admit him overnight, so we did. It was a horrible hospital. For three days no doctor came to see us. We just sat in a room with other patients, waiting for our turn, totally helpless. We saw people in complete agony and pain—even one person who looked like his insides were coming out of him. I don't know how else to explain it, but that's what I saw. And it was filthy. The food they offered us—*daal*[2] and burnt *rotis*—no one could eat it. There was no one to complain to, and no one keeping anyone accountable. After three days, I just couldn't imagine my son being treated there. So we left.

After that, at the recommendation of my youngest brother, I came here to Bhaktivedanta Hospital. When our son was admitted, the doctors treated us as though we were fam-

---

2. *Daal* is a soup made from lentils.

ily, even though we didn't even know them. Our son was placed in the 5th floor isolation ward. He was here for three days, and made a full recovery. The day he came, he said he was already halfway healed.

It was at that time that Seemi, our Spiritual Care nurse, came to meet us. She was just like a mother, like an angel. She made sure we were fed, she asked us how we were feeling, and she spoke to us about spirituality. She was so concerned about us, I felt she was the Goddess herself, or perhaps God's representative. Since that time, we have also been patients here ourselves, as have been our other son and our daughter-in-law, for minor illnesses. We would do anything for Seemi. Today, we were going to go to the village for two months, but she asked if we'd like to come here to meet you, and we were so eager to do something for her to reciprocate with all her love.

Neha: With age and with spirituality, we have learned to be more peaceful. It's amazing how we used to worry so much, and how we used to try to acquire so many things. Now, we still have no "things;" there are days when we don't even eat. But somehow, we are peaceful.

Rakesh: One of the most important lessons we learned here at this hospital is that we are not in control. I lost my job in 1995; the whole company went under. Since then, I've just been taking odd jobs here and there to somehow get by. My son also brings home some money every month.

Both of my sons are educated. My elder son did his Bachelor of Commerce, and my younger son is enrolled in his first year of a Bachelor of Arts program. The money for the education came from the odd jobs I took, and also a little shop we run out of our home from time to time. We get by. We've always adjusted our lifestyle to be able to send our kids to school.

Ever since we started believing in God, it's like I have nothing but I have everything. Seemi taught me to trust what God wants, and he will provide what I need. I know I have to enjoy or suffer the results of my actions, and God will still take care of me.

Neha: We are from *brahmana* families, but we didn't learn anything about spirituality growing up. When we learned from Seemi about the chanting of Hare Krishna, we didn't do it regularly because we didn't have the time; we were so busy. But I saw from Seemi's example that if I really wanted to, I could make the time. We could do *japa* together as a family. Now if I don't chant, I don't feel peaceful. If I don't chant my rounds, I'll wake up in the middle of the night and remember, and I'll get up to chant. Whatever I do, I try to chant while I'm doing it. We used to think that religion was for old people, but now I wish I had been chanting this *mantra* for my entire life. How much more peaceful we could have been!

Rakesh: Sometimes it's hard to chant every day and follow the dietary restrictions, but Seemi taught us that when we voluntarily make a sacrifice for Krishna, he becomes very happy. If you give him an inch, he'll give you back a mile. And people respect you when you stay true to your principles.

We just can't stop talking about Seemi. She is a true lady of God. We were always taught that we shouldn't praise people to their face, just in case they might become proud or arrogant as a result. In fact, we should criticize a person to their face, and praise them behind their back. That's how we were taught. But there's nothing bad to say about her! We call her all the time. Whatever I am today I feel is because of her. I'm finally happy—and I really feel it's because of Seemi and what she has given us.

Interview with Seemi Verma

Spiritual Care Assistant
January 14, 2014

I have been a Spiritual Care Assistant here at the Bhaktivedanta Hospital for eight, lovely years. I've just written the exam to get promoted to a Junior Officer. It was quite the journey for me to get to this point.

I was born in a family of Krishna devotees. My parents and paternal grandparents are all great devotees of Krishna. My paternal grandmother is the one who taught me to chant Hare Krishna. She was so wise, even though she wasn't educated and never learned how to read. She would always have us read to her, so many books—the *Bhagavad-gita*, the *Ramayana*, the *Bhagavatam*, and more. She was an exemplary devotee in her thoughts, words, and actions. A widow at the age of 35, she pretty much raised three boys and one girl alone. She was one amazing lady. My mother's family follows Vallabha Acarya from a different line of devotees that are not Hare Krishnas. In that group, I accepted a guru at a very young age.

✤ ✤ ✤ ✤

Family Life and Struggles

I have three sisters and two brothers. I am the eldest. We lived in a joint family system, which is common in India. A joint family is one in which all the sons of the house don't move out—after they get married, they bring their wives into their parents' home, and raise their children together there. We grew up in the same house with our two uncles, and their wives and kids. There were 15 kids in total in our house! It was wonderful. I had a great childhood. My parents loved each other a lot. We had a beautiful house and family, and a lot of love.

My father worked very hard to create his own business empire in the wedding industry, and he was extremely successful. He would provide decorations and overall event management for large weddings. My mother was beautiful and simple. We all grew up feeling secure, and with positive self-esteem. I attribute much of our happy home atmosphere to my grandmother as well. She was so spiritual. She'd be up late at night meditating, and then again in the morning she'd be very engrossed in her devotional service. She wouldn't eat before 2:30 p.m. I have vivid memories of her singing "Gopi Geet."[3] Because of her, *bhakti* is in our blood. She was quite strict, and always taught me that I should know how to look after myself. She used to teach us how to cook and sew. One of my fondest memories of us is making quilts together. Because of her training, we'd also be able to help with the business—we'd decorate the altars where people got married, the pillows, and more. Whatever my grandmother taught me, I ended up doing professionally: knitting, stitching, embroidery, and related arts. My grandmother always said we should be prepared to be mothers, and good daughters-in-law. For her, that meant being domestic experts —proficient in cooking, cleaning, sewing, raising children, and similar things. She had very high expectations of me.

My grandmother has been gone for 13 years but I remember her every single day at least once. She gave me everything—culture, memories, life skills—and she was illiterate! She gave me much more than I could ever give my kids. She died at 85. Imagine! She was a widow for 50 years.

---

[3]. A prayerful song, often recited in the holy month of *Kartik* (October—November). Its verses are derived from the *Srimad Bhagavatam*.

I did a bachelor's degree in arts, and then I started my MA, but I stopped at the age of 26 because my parents arranged my marriage. They didn't know my husband's family too well, but knew his family was of the same caste.

My husband's name is Vikram. Our wedding was a grand affair. It lasted three days, in 1990. My father really outdid himself to throw us a beautiful, extravagant celebration. To this day, people tell me they remember my wedding as one of the most enjoyable and festive events they've ever attended. We got married in my hometown in Gujarat, and three days later we came back here to Mumbai. My daughter was born in March of 1991. That same year my father-in-law passed away. At that time, we struggled greatly. Of course, we were emotionally distraught to have lost my father-in-law, but also having a new baby was overwhelming both emotionally and financially. It's hard for me not to weep when I think about how much we struggled.

For the first two years of our relationship, my husband and I got along very well. But afterwards, we didn't at all. The more I got to know him, the more I became uncomfortable. He had some bad habits I'd never even heard of before. He was also a very heavy drinker. It made me feel unsafe, especially having grown up with such a wholesome, protective father, and having such a sheltered life until that point. The contrast was glaring.

Vik would try different business ventures but one by one they'd all fail. To help out, I took on a number of odd jobs, and I opened nurseries at home. I did that for about seven years. We had another daughter, and then a son. I helped and supported my husband in every way possible. I never asked him for anything. Still, the environment at home was never peaceful; there was always tension. I was so worried about what it was doing to the children. I'd do so much for my husband, and I used to feel so upset that he'd never even acknowledge my efforts to support him and our family. My husband was never peaceful, and he never let any of us be peaceful.

That's how my life was for a while—I would only say whatever I needed to say to my husband. I'd do my duty by feeding him, making his bed, and cleaning, but I wasn't emotionally attached to him at all. Even today, I have no expectations of him. It is simply not in my destiny to take anything from this man. You know, the whole time we have been married, he has never even bought me one *sari*. Whatever nice things I owned, whether they were *saris* or jewellery, he sold them. He even sold some of my mother's jewellery. Somehow, I was able to earn enough money to buy most of it back.

Vik's parents never got along with each other. They always argued. He never saw a healthy marriage growing up; unhealthy relations between husband and wife were all he ever saw.

Vik's nature is to doubt me. He used to get angry if another man even looked at me. He used to argue with me all the time, and not even let me leave the house. Even if I were breastfeeding at home with the door closed, he'd come in and question how much I'd cover myself while breastfeeding. He'd always doubt my character and commitment.

He would get upset and torture me every time I went to visit my parents. Nothing was a discussion; everything was an argument. Even in front of my family, he'd fight so viciously with me. I never, ever, got financial, physical, or emotional support from him.

I think my dad had some concerns about my marrying Vikram. He asked me many times if I was sure. Honestly, I was just so tired of looking. I kept seeing the bios of all these men and none of them were of any interest to me. So when I saw Vik's information I just thought, "It's fine. No problem, I'll just do it." I was 25 when I got married. At that time, that was considered very old. Women would get married at 22 or 23 at the latest. Everyone used to say to my father, "How much longer will you wait to marry her off?" But he never forced me. He wanted me to marry the right person. Still, I was feeling guilty that he really had to endure so much from so many people. I didn't want to cause him more stress so I just got married. But, nothing about me and Vik matched. I went from a life where I never worried about anything financially, to one where I'd sometimes wonder how we'd eat.

One of the odd jobs I once held was helping sew the falls[4] on *saris*. There was a lady who used to sell beautiful, heavy *saris* who lived a floor beneath us. For all the *saris* she'd sell, I'd sew on the fall for her. I used to stay up really late—until 1:30 a.m. or so—just to finish on time. Then I'd wake up early, get the kids ready for school, pack lunches, and be at work at the *sari* store at 10 a.m. I'd get home by 7 or 8 p.m. Vik used to suspect that maybe I was having an affair with the lady's husband. He'd get mad if I ever even spoke to him. I used to be so scared of my husband. I'd barely even talk to him; I'd just answer questions if he asked. He fought with me so much about this man. One day, I spoke up. I said, "You don't allow me to leave! I took a job *in our building* to make you happy. No matter what I do, you fight with me!"

And then he hit me. Hard. It was the first time he laid a hand on me. I was shocked, and angry.

"You're not working!" I said to him. "So *I am*. You *know*

---

4. A "fall" is a strip of cloth sewn at the bottom of a *sari* to help its pleats fall nicely.

I'm faithful to you. I work for nothing from morning to night, and still, you want to argue with me?"

I was so hurt. So I left. I couldn't handle it anymore. I had thought before about ending my life, but that day, I was determined.

I walked to the nearest train station. It was about 7:30 p.m., and quite dark outside. As usual, the train station was bustling with tea and book vendors, businessmen and women, mothers with their children, porters, and beggars of all kinds asking for money. Yet I felt completely alone. Thousands of commuters passed me by, scurrying to catch the train to Borivali, and no one noticed me inching closer to the tracks. I was standing on the first of four platforms, where there would be a train going to Borivali from Churchgate.

"When the next train comes, just jump. Just one small leap, and it will all be over," I told myself.

Then a train arrived, and the speed of it startled me. I fell backwards into the crowd. For a moment, I considered turning around and running as far away from the tracks as I could. The train stopped, opened its doors, and heaps of commuters walked past me, over me, into me, just shoving me aside to board or exit the train. Not one person stopped to help me. My resolve to jump returned.

The next train arrived, and again, it startled me, and I didn't jump. Three attempts later, I fell to the ground and cried, feeling like a failure in my life, and in the attempt to end my life. After about an hour of crying alone in the station, I stood up, and, feeling dejected, walked home. I dreaded going back home. At the same time, when I did, I remember never being happier to see my kids.

That was one of the lowest points in my life. Somehow, I kept going. For the kids' sake, I vowed never to try to take my life again. I shudder when I think about the impact it would have had on them.

The kids grew up fast, living in our house. Today, my daughters Rekha and Anshu are 23 and 20, and my son, Aarav is 14. They all have a decent relationship with their father. They're extremely mature and want to believe the best in him. Thankfully, all my kids are well situated today, and have good heads on their shoulders. Aarav is in the eighth grade, one daughter is doing a Bachelors degree in Engineering, and the other a Bachelor of Education.

Whatever we have is from my earnings. I buy Vikram's clothes. He doesn't help out with any of the housework. I used to feel sometimes that he lived only to disturb me.

In 2012, I lost my mother. It was devastating. She had a problem with her lungs, and a brain hemorrhage. My father is currently a healthy 78-year-old. He knows a little bit about my situation at home, but I don't really tell him much. He can see that I'm not that happy. Thankfully, my sisters are all good—great families, good financial situations. My sisters know about my troubles; I couldn't keep it from them. My youngest sister and I are particularly close—I tell her everything.

Today, Vikram and I are in a better place, but it took us a long time to get here.

❦ ❦ ❦ ❦

Meeting People from the Bhaktivedanta Hospital

One day, I attended a relative's engagement party. As it turned out, this relative of mine was getting married to the cousin of a devotee from the Chowpatty temple, and I met her at this party. She had a clinic where Dr. Komal Dalal was giving regular lectures. She invited me to come, but I wasn't interested. I was so disturbed and unhappy, and in a very poor financial state. I felt that I needed to focus on my life, and not on spirituality, which was not helpful for me. Everyone would tell me all the time that I should worship so many different personalities—Sai Baba, Devi, Shivji—and I used to do it. I'd do everything that people told me. But it wasn't really from the heart and I didn't feel like it was doing anything for me. It was more ritualistic than anything. I was turned off by all the temples that were always asking for money, as if spirituality and peace were things to be purchased. It was so hard to find legitimate devotees. So, when this devotee was inviting me, I really wasn't interested; I just figured that this, like everything else, would be an attempt to take my money. Every time she invited me, I continued to make excuses. I kept thinking, "What's in it for her?" I gave her my number, and she stayed in touch. Every once in a while, she'd invite me again.

One day, I finally relented and I went. That day, my life totally changed. I was completely blown away. There was such purity in the speaker and all the people present. I couldn't believe it. I went for three weeks in a row, and on that third visit I was convinced that *bhakti* was for me. Dr. Dalal was incredible—she held my hand and lovingly guided me through the course she was administering, called "The Journey of Self Discovery," named after a book by Srila Prabhupada. I found myself becoming so engaged—I'd spend hours preparing for each class. The philosophy was so clear to me, unlike any other temple or philosophy I was exposed to. It was clear, scientific, and also heartfelt. I had a lot questions, and the devotees always patiently answered all of them, and made me feel comfortable to ask more, and to authentically address all my doubts. They were so loving and kind. They could see that I was struggling in life, so some of them started to encourage me to meditate every day by chanting one round of Hare Krishna, which would take approximately seven minutes. I'd resist and tell them I had no time. No one ever pressured me. Eventually, I started chanting one round once in a while. I realized that I did have the time, if I really wanted. I didn't tell them that I'd have a two-hour nap every day! The kids were so small, and I'd help them with their homework, and then take naps—no matter what, I always had time for a nap! Still, I stuck to one round, and that soon became daily.

Through the course and the chanting, I suddenly felt connected to my grandmother again. Everything I was learning was what my grandmother used to teach me growing up. At some point in my life, I became so distraught that I thought that happiness could be found elsewhere, outside of *bhakti*. But I didn't find happiness anywhere. I realized, in that class, that happiness for me is in *bhakti*, and that I had it all along. It doesn't mean your problems go away, but it means that you can cope and have perspective.

Unfortunately, my husband didn't like that I was going to these gatherings, and he eventually forbade me to go. I was devastated. Every two or three months, I'd make up an excuse and go. I'd also try to attend the counselling meetings here at the hospital. If someone would like to formally accept a mentor or counsellor here, there are mandatory meetings to attend. The problem was they were so late at night—from 8 p.m. to 10 p.m. I had very nosy and judgmental neighbours, who made atrocious comments if they saw me ever coming in late. They would make terrible assumptions, and it would anger my husband greatly, so I had to stop attending.

❖ ❖ ❖

Gopal's Garden

In 2002, we were looking for a school for my son Aarav to attend. Dr. Dalal encouraged me to apply for Gopal's Garden, the school affiliated with Bhaktivedanta Hospital. The tuition was cheaper, which was very appealing. But more appealing than that, it was a school that was teaching the students about *bhakti*. I was able to convince my husband to let Aarav apply, on the grounds that it was the most affordable. It felt amazing that my son would be introduced to *bhakti*, with no argument from my husband, and that I could actually afford to send him. During Aarav's application process, we had a few interviews with some of the school administrators. They told us that in order for a child to have a proper education in *bhakti*, it is integral to have a devotional atmosphere at home as well: one that was peaceful, and conducive to spirituality. Maybe they could tell that I was a little nervous about being able to maintain such an atmosphere at home, so they encouraged me to rejoin the counsellor program for guidance. It was perfect—Vikram couldn't object now, because I could frame it as a complement to Aarav's schooling! I went regularly and joined Dr. Dalal's group, and she became my official counsellor. To this day, I can't adequately express my gratitude for her. Her words have so much power, and she always helps me be peaceful. She is inspirational. My husband started to attend a course, too, because the school highly encouraged parents to attend the courses and meetings at the hospital so they could understand what their kids were learning at school. In this way, we could try to implement spiritual principles at home as well. Within six months, I was committed. My husband wasn't, but he started to come to the temple once in a while, and to some of the other programs at the hospital. He started to understand that the people of this hospital are good people, doing good work. He recognized that they were a pious group. In time, he also joined me in counselling meetings. It felt like a miracle.

This was a time in my life when things really started to look up. My financial struggles were slowly going away. I started to run a nursery at home. Twenty to thirty kids were coming to my house to learn, and it was wonderful! I didn't have much experience, but I loved kids a lot. I loved serving them. I never felt bad about cleaning up after them; I'd do it with love. In this way, my income started to increase little by little. I started to think, "Wow, Krishna is helping me!" and I started to chant 16 rounds of Hare Krishna, which is the recommended amount for committed *bhakti* practitioners. In total, it takes about two hours. I also tried to improve my overall *bhakti* routine. I'd give the nursery kids *prasadam* to eat, and I used to feed them on my lap. It brought so much joy to my heart. At first, they had a lot of separation anxiety from their parents and they would cry. But after some time, they'd cry to their parents to be with me on the weekends! The parents would tell me that their children would say, "Can you cook the way she cooks?" What a joy.

Then, in 2003, our landlord decided to sell our home, and I had to move. My entire nursery program had to close because I moved quite far. For a year in the new house, I tried to start another nursery but there were just not enough kids in that neighbourhood. I was very tense. I went back to taking odd jobs here and there. Over the next three years, I tried a few times to restart a nursery, but it just never worked out. I was wondering what to do—how to earn money and also how to pass my time. Eventually, I started to understand that both situations were blessings from

Krishna—when I was comfortable financially, and when I was struggling financially.

※ ※ ※ ※

A Vacancy at the Hospital

It was then, in 2006, while I was struggling to keep a nursery afloat, that Dr. Dalal told me about a vacancy here in the Spiritual Care department. I told her I wasn't interested—I had absolutely no medical background, and I wasn't interested in being around illness. Even the thought of blood made me feel nauseous. Dr. Dalal told me that for this particular job, I'd be trained in some medical basics but that the job was only to befriend and speak to patients. I still had my reservations, but because of our dire financial situation, I thought I'd at least apply and learn more about the position.

I had an interview with Dr. Vivek Shanbhag. He asked me frankly if I'd be comfortable working in a hospital. I told him that I couldn't bear to see any open wounds, or burns, or anything else too traumatizing. He told me that he wouldn't be able to fully protect me from seeing such things, but that he could arrange that I'd never be assigned to the ICU. He also told me that the main service was seeing patients who've already been treated, and therefore wouldn't have open wounds. We both agreed that I could start working here on a trial basis.

I hated it. I couldn't handle all the sickness. The burn victims. The accident victims. I'd get dizzy and queasy. On top of that, I had a very long commute, and before that I wasn't even used to ever leaving the house! And then, within my first few weeks here, the terrorist attacks happened in the Mumbai train system. All I saw were burn victims. I couldn't believe it; it was horrifying.

But, when I saw the devotees here working hard and caring so nicely for those patients, I couldn't help but be inspired. As much as I couldn't stand the sight of all these atrocities, I also couldn't tear myself away. I had to stay and help. And I was in the best company—the people here are so wonderful and I wanted their association. They inspired me to want to stay and help, to assist them and to offer services similar to the ones they were offering. Even in the temples, I didn't find such pure-hearted people as those who work here. I received so much support and care from them, and I became very attached to them. I was starving for love and care, and here I was getting it so easily. As soon as I felt a little stronger and built up again, it was very natural to want to pay it forward. I was in a job that was literally paying me to be loving! To be a version of myself I had lost for so long. I realized that all this love was in me to give, and I could make a real difference just by befriending patients. This job made me a better mother, friend, sister, daughter, and even wife. It has filled me up so completely.

I became hooked. And here I am, eight years later.

After one month of working here I got over my fears and was able to work in the ICU and with wounded patients. My job is to help and to provide spiritual support to others, but I can't begin to explain all the ways this hospital has helped me grow. My job is simply to pay it forward. I recently attended a seminar here on Empathic Listening. I know that in India, courses like this are not offered regularly at hospitals. But here at Bhaktivedanta Hospital, they are constantly teaching us the skills to become better caregivers, and they are skills I can apply in my personal life as well. Everyone here is doing so many great things. Dr. Dalal travels the world to give seminars about holistic care. When she tells me about her experiences I feel really inspired. She taught me a lot about how to deal with patients suffering from substance abuse or addiction.

At home, my husband didn't always allow me to go to the temple. But just by coming to work, I was in such a devotional atmosphere—I was earning and learning at the same time.

※ ※ ※ ※

Committing to *Bhakti*

In my first year of joining the hospital, I attended a number of seminars and had the good fortune to meet some wonderful people. There were always programs or festivals to attend. Slowly, I started to understand how herculean this mission is, to provide holistic care to people, including those who couldn't afford to be treated. When I saw the love, time, and energy people invested in this hospital, I started to understand that I was a part of something huge and very special. In time, I also started to see the importance of the Spiritual Care department, and I became overwhelmed with gratitude that I got to be a part of it.

I also started to learn more about Radhanath Swami, the guiding force and inspiration of this hospital. He travels around the world, sharing *bhakti* with hundreds of thousands of people. People around the world long for his personal attention, but just by his creating this department all the patients here get access to his love. It is deeply personal. He has such a huge heart. I feel like all we are doing is distributing his love. People come here and then miracles happen in their lives. They give up unhealthy addictions, they mend relationships—they experience so much positivity and become inspired from within. So many of them become more spiritual, regardless of what religion they practice. People get out of depression when they come here. So many people have started chanting Hare Krishna as a result of this association; even staff members, like me. We join the mentorship system and receive an abundance of love and care, and so many also take up the chanting, or rosary, or equivalent. This place is mystical. And for me, I feel like I'm hopefully being of service to Radhanath Swami by working here. He can't meet with each patient, but still, his extreme care is pouring down on every single patient because of this Spiritual Care department that he conceptualized and created. It has saved *my* life, what to speak of the patients!

I went from being quite skeptical of spirituality, to being fully committed. It helped that no one has ever pressured me. I always have been, and continue to be, encouraged to ask questions, express doubts, and really make *bhakti* my own.

As I mentioned earlier, I already had another guru. I didn't even know what it meant to have a guru. I heard somewhere that one should only accept one husband and one guru. So, I told myself I'd continue to try and progress in *bhakti*, but that I just wouldn't accept an official guru. One day, Dr. Dalal asked me if I wanted to officially take on a guru and become an official disciple in the *bhakti* tradition. My heart changed—I just knew that Radhanath Swami is my guru, and that he always will be. In 2012, Radhanath Swami formally accepted me as his disciple.

I have never spoken to Radhanath Swami directly, but I don't have to. I feel directly and intimately connected to him through this service. He does so much for the entire world, sacrifices so much—this is a small way to give back and help him distribute Srila Prabhupada's compassion.

Growing as a Caregiver

I used to be so afraid of death. Even if a relative or someone I knew passed away, I'd not visit the family—it just scared me too much.

Now, my biggest and most important service is end-of-life care. This service is so fulfilling because I feel that God has made me his instrument, to help people at this most important moment of life—the time they are leaving their bodies. At this critical time, I am chanting the names of God for them, and helping them leave with dignity. It's what I'm meant to do. Now, when I hear about death, I *run* to be by the patient's side.

Param

All of us have developed the habit of writing down our favourite patient stories. There are so many that inspire us. One man, Param, used to come regularly for dialysis. He was 63 years old at the time, and always so positive. He had started the dialysis in 2002, and I met him in 2006 when I joined the hospital. When we first started talking, he began to express interest in spirituality, so one day, by *rickshaw*, I delivered him some *bhakti* books called the *Srimad Bhagavatam* and the *Chaitanya Caritamrita*. He loved to read; he would read for an average of six hours every day! He completed the entire multivolume *Srimad Bhagavatam* before I did! Then he started reading the mammoth *Chaitanya Caritamrita*, and completed that too! Next, I gave him the biography of Srila Prabhupada. He read that, and then the *Srimad Bhagavatam* again. He would spend all his free time reading— no TV or anything else. He didn't just read—he studied. He took copious notes. He was becoming more and more peaceful.

In 2008 he started to chant four rounds of Hare Krishna every day. After six months, he started to cut down on his meat intake. He told me that it was customary in his family to feed guests meat, so he'd cook it and sometimes eat it, too. I felt he was really inclined to become a vegetarian, and just needed a nudge. I even felt like he was asking for one. I told him that in Indian culture, sharing sweets is customary—not meat. That's all I said, and he gave up meat completely. We talked about our great fortune to have access to these wonderful spiritual books. I told him that I felt that Srila Prabhupada must be so happy with him, for reading his books so thoroughly, and also now applying the principles in his life. I told him he was the recipient of so much kindness from God. He told me later that his guests started to understand that no meat would be available at his house, and they were fine with it.

He really, truly believed in each verse he read. He loved the hospital, he loved all the festivals, and he loved all the Spiritual Care nurses. He said that this kidney disease was a blessing, because without it he wouldn't have come to Bhaktivedanta Hospital.

He passed away three years ago. He left behind a loving wife and two daughters. His youngest daughter used to come here regularly to drop off her father. You can see on her face how sweet she is. I stay in touch with her—her name is Shilpa. She is now chanting, and both she and her mother came for the "Journey of Self Discovery" seminar. Since taking that course, they have been totally fixed in *bhakti*. They are also now in the counsellor system. They live here on Mira Road.

My Life Today

When Jayapataka Swami was a patient here, I used to frequently visit him. No visitors were allowed except for us. Every day I would go for *Ratha Seva*,[5] and the Swami would speak to me personally all the time. Even to this day, if we ever see each other, he recognizes me right away. He used to always ask us to read patient stories to him; he loved them all. I would speak in Hindi, and someone would translate for me. He was here again recently for a checkup. Every time he comes, he says, "Who can tell me a story?" And he always lectures on these stories too! Radhanath Swami says that even he doesn't know as many stories about the hospital as Jayapataka Swami!

I felt so happy to speak with him. The soul becomes happy when associated with anything spiritual. The truth is, there is absolutely no satisfaction, or lasting happiness in anything material. What we have at this hospital is so rare. I'm not sure how I got so lucky.

My life completely changed by meeting the people from this hospital. My family changed. When Aarav joined Gopal's Garden everything got even better. And he wouldn't have joined this school if we weren't having so many financial difficulties.

All of my difficulties led me here. It is written in our scriptures that when one is very beautiful, it is easy to become proud. I was. I was beautiful, and I was proud. My eldest daughter looks just like me when I was her age. But with

---

5. Every day at Bhaktivedanta Hospital, a makeshift altar ("Ratha") with the deity of Jagannath is wheeled to each patient's room, to give him or her the opportunity to offer the deity a flower. The service of taking the altar from room to room is called "Ratha Seva."

my husband, all my pride went away. I never felt beautiful. I don't think I'm so beautiful now, but I was when I was younger. With everything that I've gone through, I feel I've got no pride left. And to be honest, this has been a wonderful catalyst in my spiritual life. In fact, all my suffering has been a wonderful catalyst. Everything has been the sweet plan of the Lord; even the hard times. In the end, I'm grateful for all of it.

By working at Bhaktivedanta Hospital, I can see that everyone is suffering. Every single person in this world is suffering mentally and emotionally, if not physically. People come here with such horrible stories, so much sadness, and it makes me realize that suffering is just the regular human condition. It's a feature of the material world, there's no escaping it. People come here for their physical needs but they are also emotionally hurting. That's why this hospital is so special—patients get treated for everything, emotionally, socially, spiritually, and physically.

My daughter is now engaged to be married, and I have been supporting her financially, mentally, and emotionally. I'm so pleased with my daughter and her fiancé. They are both ambitious and humble. I never want them to experience the same financial difficulties that we did. Her fiancé comes from a very kind, and well-off family. They have their own business, and they're also very good people. And they're not proud of what they have.

I always prayed my girls would get married early, as long as it was to good men from good families. I just wanted them to be secure, healthy, and happy, as any parent does.

As of late, things have also been getting better with my husband. Together, we attended seminars at the hospital put on by a teacher named Sukhavaha *Devi*. From her, we learned skills like effective listening, communication, and expression of feelings. She did about twelve sessions with us, gave us homework, and we would share our experiences with each other about how we were trying to apply her teachings both at work and at home. I used to victimize myself—"He's not helping me, he's not treating me right." But it took me a while to understand that I had to work on myself, too.

This hospital has given me so much. Now, whenever I'm not here at the hospital, I miss it. I just want to serve more and more.

☙ ☙ ☙

RB: Seemi's daughter was scheduled to have a formal engagement ceremony about a month after this conversation. Seemi lovingly and enthusiastically invited me, but I was unable to attend. We spoke again, a few days after the ceremony. Our conversation is transcribed below.

Oh, the engagement ceremony for my daughter was perfect! It was all arranged by my future son-in-law's family. They gifted her with many beautiful *saris* and jewellery. It was such a festive occasion. The food, the entertainment—everything was perfect. My husband had never seen anything like it. He loved it. My daughter is marrying into a great family that genuinely loves her very much. You always worry as a parent—"Will they keep my daughter happy? Will they give her any trouble? How will they be? Are they good or not?" But yesterday at the engagement, I didn't question any of that for one moment. They love her so much. That fear is gone from our minds. She will be well treated and very happy.

My husband was very happy, too! That day felt like some sort of arrival—a milestone. We are in a better place in our relationship, and we were able to afford a beautiful celebration for our daughter. For the engagement, it was important to me to go all out. I saved as much money as I could, so I could spend it on the festivities. I really wanted this to be the perfect day for my daughter, and it was.

Growing up, I never had any financial difficulties. It was only after marriage that I really struggled. Thankfully, it will be the opposite for my daughter. We struggled when she was young, but now, thanks to her education and also marrying into a good family, she will be okay. My husband had tears in his eyes, because he could see how lucky his daughter is. He said to her, "Your mother-in-law loves you very much. You are very lucky. Give her all love and respect, always." As he was speaking, he was stroking her hair and face. He had never done anything like that before. "You are our princess, marrying a prince," he said. "They all really love you."

Then he looked at me and said, "Seemu, I never thought our daughter would leave us so soon, and that she'd get something so good. I feel like this is a dream."

For the first time in a very long time, I could see and appreciate that my husband actually has a very soft heart, and I felt affection and happiness with him.

I wouldn't be here today without having access to Srila Prabhupada's books. It still amazes me that I have to read them *for my job*. I'm so lucky. It wasn't always easy for me to read at home, but I always get to do it at work! It's my job, and my growth all in one. Earning and learning, together. Srila Prabhupada brought me here to learn, not teach. And now, by his grace, I get to pay it forward. I often think about that day I almost ended my life. Can you imagine? Now, being here, at the Bhaktivedanta Hospital, and seeing the progress my family has made by the grace of God—there is no greater gift.

Interview with Dr. Venkata Ramanan

Director of Projects and Program—Share Your Care
January 22, 2014

⚜ ⚜ ⚜ ⚜

The Beginnings

One day many years ago, I was walking home from the train station, and it started to rain heavily. I was just around the corner from home, but it was raining so heavily that I ducked inside the Mira Road temple for shelter. I bumped into Dr. Sankhe, who was also seeking shelter from the rain. He was a friendly acquaintance at the time; we didn't know each other very well. I had seen him at the temple occasionally though I wasn't a serious practitioner of *bhakti* back then. We started to chat, and he asked where I was working. I was working with a US multinational that manufactured floppy discs and other electronic items. I didn't mind the job, but I despised the commute. In fact, I was considering selling my flat and moving to a smaller city because the craziness of Mumbai was really starting to get to me. I felt it was really becoming a rat race; no matter how successful I could be in my career, I'd still just be a rat, like everyone else, being out of my flat for up to 16 hours a day, without spending much time with my wife and children.

I was expressing my frustration to Dr. Sankhe that day, and he said, "Moving is not the solution to all your problems; if you're not happy in one place, you're likely not to be happy in another. You have to feel happy inside."

In hindsight, that is clear. In the moment, it felt like a jolt.

"We're in the process of building a team for our hospital, just down the road from here," he said. "Maybe we can talk about some potential opportunities for you."

The prospect of a change, without having to sell my flat and uproot my family was very compelling. And, I would be able to work with Dr. Sankhe, who was well respected in the community, and I could work in a spiritual environment. I was really attracted to *bhakti* and to the devotees, so this was an enticing proposition.

For four months, I continued working for the other company, and I'd consult for Bhaktivedanta Hospital once a week. I slowly started to increase my time at Bhaktivedanta, and decrease my time at the other job, until I was at the hospital four days a week and one day at the other job. My boss at the other company asked me what it was about this hospital that was so attractive to me.

"I can't explain it," I said. "Come with me tomorrow and meet the team."

I brought him here to the hospital, and after he met some of the staff and saw what we were doing here, he said to me, "I am not going to come between you and this place; it's phenomenal. You are at liberty to leave, whenever you're ready."

Any trace of obligation I felt towards the other organization vanished with those words. To this day, I am friends with my old boss and colleagues, and they've even donated a significant amount to the hospital.

༈ ༈ ༈ ༈

My Role

I have been associated with this hospital for the last 17 years. At the very beginning, I was leading a number of the non-medicinal aspects of the hospital—mainly in Administration, Human Resources, and Finance. As we grew, we hired people to look after Administration and HR, and I now sit with the Finance group. I'm focused more on strategic planning for various projects and fundraising. Our fundraising efforts are for the operations of the hospital, and to try to cover care for people who can't afford it. For people who cannot afford medical care, we provide concessions typically in the range of 30-50%, and in many cases, for free.

In the initial years, we were just getting on our feet, understanding the needs of a hospital, and trying to build a foundation. In 2002, we decided we were ready to do more outreach activities. This is when the Community Outreach group began to take shape. One of the roles of this group is to screen potential candidates for free cataract surgery. We have performed about 5,000 free cataract surgeries to date, which means the Community Outreach group has screened over 50,000 candidates. It's no small job![6]

꙳ ꙳ ꙳ ꙳

Tiny Miracles

I'm not a clinical staff member, so I'm not always exposed to the miracles that happen with patients, but I hear about them daily. Still, even here, within Finance, there have been so many little miracles. I feel like it's almost a pastime of Lord Krishna's—to compel us to lean on him, and show us he's listening.

There's one example that comes to mind. It was the end of September 2001, and I was travelling in Pune to do some benchmarking with other hospitals. Before I left, I had instructed the members of the team that 8 lakh rupees [Rs. 800,000] were to remain untouched, as we had to make a loan payment on October 1 of 7 lakhs. On the 30th of

---

[6]. At the time of editing (2025) this number has increased to 10,000+ free cataract surgeries per year.

September, I returned from my trip and was told that one of the higher-ups had used *all* the funds for another emergency purpose. *All of them.* There was nothing left for essential payments, including salaries. I was flabbergasted. I had even issued some post-dated cheques. I was so upset, and completely worried. The funds were used for a legitimate purpose, but now I was in a terrible situation.

Usually, I leave the office at 7 or 8 p.m., but that day I left at 5:30 p.m. I was so disturbed. As I left, I offered my respects to the deity of Srila Prabhupada at the main entrance of the hospital.

"Please, Srila Prabhupada," I said with folded hands. "Please bail us out of this situation. I am fully dependent on you."

I went home, feeling physically ill. At about 8 p.m., I got a call. It was Hrishikesh.

"Hare Krishna," he said in his usual upbeat tone.

"*Haribol*[7], *Prabhu*," I said, feeling dejected.

"For two years, we have been fostering a relationship with a potential donor," said Hrishikesh. "He had indicated that he wanted to donate to the hospital, but after some time, we lost hope. But just today, my secretary in Ahmedabad told me that this donor just sent a check for 7.25 lakhs, and asked that someone pick up the cheque tomorrow. Could you please find someone to pick it up?"

I wasn't sure if I heard correctly.

"What? How ... when ... what?" I was thrilled. I was *so* thrilled. This was the *exact* amount that was required to clear the loan.

Time and time again, Srila Prabhupada and Lord Krishna

---

7. *Haribol* is a common greeting among *bhakti* practitioners, meaning, "Chant the name of Lord Hari!" ("Hari" is another name of Lord Krishna.)

have shown us that they're listening. I believe they are reciprocating with the sincerity and sacrifice of the founding doctors of this hospital. This hospital is founded on their sacrifices and extreme difficulties. This is one of the driving forces for me; this is what makes me feel loyal.

Interview with Vaidehi Nawathe

Chief Dietician
January 30, 2014

When I found out that the Bhaktivedanta Hospital is a vegetarian hospital, I couldn't believe it. I grew up in a traditional Hindu *brahmana* family, where eating meat was prohibited. From a compassion and nonviolence perspective, I was a vegetarian, but as I studied nutrition, I also understood the negative physiological effects of eating meat. I'd always hoped that I could work for a hospital that didn't serve meat, but I knew that was an unrealistic hope. And then magically, I found out about this hospital in 1998, applied, and got a job as a dietician!

I didn't know who Srila Prabhupada was until I started working here. Since I started, it's become clear to me that this building, this vision, this purpose—it's all coming from Srila Prabhupada, and that Radhanath Swami is carrying it out. I strongly and confidently believe that we, the staff at Bhaktivedanta Hospital, have been placed here to be servants of the patients, and that we are being managed by Srila Prabhupada. What I've realized, and what I teach my staff, is that we must serve our patients as if they are guests in our home. I ask my staff to go out of their way not only to give their patients as much knowledge as they need about treatment and prevention, but also to do so with a genuine personal touch.

The *bhakti* way of living resonates with everyone, regardless of religion. It's a way of life. In 2012, I was invited to speak as a dietician on a television show for three episodes. The response was tremendous, and they continue to air those episodes regularly. As a result, I wrote a column for *The Times of India* for one year, which they asked me to continue. They also asked me if I'd be interested in writing a book of articles because so many people were inquiring about this column. I never imagined something like that would happen to me!

❧ ❧ ❧ ❧

Lifestyle Choices and *Bhakti*

Bhakti-yoga is a way of life, and of course diet is a huge component of one's lifestyle.

In *bhakti*, we have a concept about the modes of material nature, namely goodness, passion, and ignorance. Everything can be placed into one of these categories; time of day, behaviours, music, association, and more. The goal is to stay in the mode of goodness, and ultimately transcend the material modes altogether and attain true love for God. There are also foods in the mode of goodness, passion, or ignorance. Foods in goodness like breads, milk, fruits, and vegetables are healthy, and they have positive effects on the body and mind. Foods in the mode of passion are spicier and can create some irritation or unrest in the body and mind. Foods in ignorance, like meat and fish, cause harm to others, and cause distress and discomfort in the body and mind. At a certain age, our bodies tend to reject or have problems with foods in the modes of passion or ignorance. Extra spices, including even onions and garlic, create an imbalance of all the resources we have in the body. Over time, this creates an overarching negative energy in the body. From a spiritual perspective, foods in the modes of passion and ignorance do not bring about peace of mind. What we eat genuinely affects our consciousness, and our ability to have peace of mind and to connect to God. Foods in the mode of goodness are best. The *bhakti* texts also teach that we should lovingly offer our food to Lord Krishna before eating it ourselves, just like we might feed an elder, or someone we love and respect, before we feed ourselves. In this way, when we eat, we are consuming God's grace, and any of the *karma* related to the food disappears. For example, we are also killing vegetables when we eat them, and therefore incur the *karma* for doing so, that is, unless we first offer it with love to God. Then, the act of eating that food becomes *karma*-free.

Growing up, my father always used to offer our food to God before we ate, but it wasn't until I came here that I really understood this concept of eating food offered to God, or *prasadam*, as such food is called in Sanskrit. All patients here receive food in the mode of goodness—food without meat, fish, eggs, garlic, and onions. All patients here love the food. Even heavy meat eaters express their surprise at how tasty the meals are, and even tell me they feel a change in their temperament. Every day, at least one patient tells me they'd like to continue this diet at home. This kind of change of heart is a reflection of *prasadam*; food has a tremendous effect on the consciousness.

When I joined the hospital, I thought that garlic was good to prescribe for certain ailments. But I've found that other things are equally effective, like cinnamon, for example.

I don't expect my patients to become students of *bhakti* philosophy, nor do I ever want to impose any spiritual values on them. But it's my duty to help them understand the physical consequences of eating all types of food, both healthy and unhealthy. Then, it's up to my patients to decide what to do. It's the same with alcohol. People give me thousands of excuses as to why they drink. If I just tell a patient to stop smoking or drinking, it won't work. But when healthcare providers give a full, fact-based picture—like if I talk to patients about how smoking and drinking affect the liver, for example—about 20% of patients come back and ask for help to stop. I usually advise people to cut down alcohol or cigarettes gradually, as opposed to all at once; in my experience, this is more effective.

In *bhakti*, everything we do in our lives is an art. This includes cooking and eating. Gratitude is of utmost importance when eating; we have to feel grateful that we've been given this meal. Similarly, the emotions we experience while cooking and serving out the food are also extremely important, as they have an effect on the body and even the consciousness of the eater. If one is agitated, angry, or disturbed while cooking, then it will have negative effects on the body, and then those negative emotions are passed on to the eater.

I believe that the root cause of so many diseases is poor food choices. The number of cancer patients is steadily increasing. We see people as young as 20 dying of heart attacks. We never used to believe that this was possible. We always thought that heart attacks were for middle-aged people with high cholesterol. But food choices affect all areas of the body, even in young bodies.

Whether or not one is a follower of *bhakti*, it is common knowledge that a vegetarian diet is better for health. A carnivorous diet can drop the PH level of our stomachs to a dangerous level. Our delicate lining is being exposed to high levels of acid due to the presence of meat in the stomach. Meat may get digested, but along with that, the body's healthy tissues and cells will also be digested. This all creates damage to the stomach lining. Additionally, putrefaction of meat takes place due to high fat content. And, the lack of fibre in meat delays the transit time in the human intestines, which are much longer than in those belonging to living entities meant to be carnivorous. This disrupts the digestion process.

When you are driving a car, you will see a signal when the petrol is running low. If you ignore it, the car will stop working. It won't even drive you across the street. It will stop. If it's a diesel vehicle, and you fill it with regular fuel, then it won't work—it's the wrong type of fuel. Similarly, humans need proteins, fats, and carbohydrates; it is our petrol. Instead, people feed their bodies diesel petrol, consisting of excessive alcohol, high fats, and meat. I'm filling the tank, but with the wrong type of fuel. So my body is bound to stop working. How? Maybe a constant cold, maybe some hair loss, maybe dark circles under the eyes, maybe a lack of sound sleep, maybe constipation. These are basic things for which no one goes to a doctor. But these things shouldn't be ignored. Otherwise, they can turn into bigger problems. And then, with time, more serious diseases will follow. What makes me sad is that these diseases can be prevented.

Another common piece of advice I give my patients is to have regular meal times. Everyone has their own bodily schedules. Perhaps one person's insulin levels peak at 12 p.m., and mine at 1 p.m. This is because of the routine we have developed. I advise my patients to respect and follow their own biological clocks. That is the basis of treating any disease—listen to your body's signals. Small things—muscle pain, the common cold—the root cause of these bodily signals is often negative feelings. It is absolutely fundamental to treat oneself holistically—body, mind, and soul. Of course, medicine is required from time to time, but sometimes it simply suppresses symptoms.

If we manage our diet properly, we can better manage our existing diseases, prevent others, and even reverse diseases. I've seen heart issues, diabetes, and even the early stages of cancer be reversed by healthy eating.

Even though I'm a dietician, I don't only speak to my patients about what to eat and what not to eat. I also discuss overall lifestyle. Sleep times, sleeping and eating patterns, levels of activity—if these things are managed positively and practically, we can more often than not achieve our health goals.

For people who tend to be physically inactive, like businesspeople that sit behind a desk all day, six hours of sleep is sufficient—maximum seven. Of course, this can vary by age and other factors, but this is true for most adults. Sleeping at the right time is also important. Sleeping at 4 a.m. and waking up at 11 may still be seven hours of sleep but it is not good for the body. We should try to be in bed by 10:30 p.m. at the latest. To be honest, 8:30 p.m. is ideal, but I recognize that is not realistic for most. Based on what I've seen, going to bed at 10:30 p.m. and rising by 4:30 a.m. is the perfect schedule. Having breakfast within two hours of waking up is also important. Plain warm water is good, or lemon and honey, or aloe vera to boost the system.

We should try not to eat anything 2-3 hours before bed. Actually, after sunset the system slows down. By 8 or 9 p.m., the organs begin their detoxification process; they start working quite hard. The liver, heart, and kidneys work to keep the body clean, so if you put food in the body during that time, the detoxification process gets slowed down or hampered. How does the body communicate this to you? There are a few signs. For example, you may not be able to wake up without an alarm. If you are in strong health, your biological clock will wake you up naturally. Secondly, if you find yourself snoozing your alarm a lot, that likely means your body needs more rest, which is also not a good sign. If you find you're dragging yourself out of bed each day and you're irritable, this is often your body telling you that it's working too hard.

Working at Bhaktivedanta Hospital

Our mission here is to serve with devotion. Along with professionalism, a touch of spirituality is key in order to connect with the soul. This is not just something I've read or heard about; I am experiencing it here daily.

It's been 16 years since I started working here, and, externally, my job appears quite routine. Every day, I make my rounds, talk to patients, write prescriptions, and counsel patients on their dietary choices. Once, a senior manager asked me if I ever get bored.

I replied, "On my days off, I think of excuses to come here anyway. Even on my days off, I'll occasionally drop by. This job is not a burden. It's not boring or mechanical. I learn something new every day from patients. As much as I try to give, I receive so much more. I get to make a difference in patients' lives, and they make a difference in mine too."

Interview with Dr. Nanasaheb Memane
Head of Ayurveda Department
February 3, 2014

I became a Hare Krishna devotee in 1999, when I was in my second year of my Bachelor of Ayurveda, Medicine and Surgery [BAMS] degree. Mr. Praveen Muley, who is currently a member of the hospital's administrative team, was a monk at the time. He was coming to my school in Nasik to give classes on spirituality. I attended them and became inspired by the philosophy, and also by his peaceful and wise demeanor. I developed a friendship with him. He was the one who inspired me to pursue my Masters degree. After he left the monastery and got married, he accepted a job at the hospital as the Deputy Director, and soon after he contacted me to see if I'd be interested in joining. He described the hospital as a holistic care facility, in need of an Ayurveda department. So, right after I completed my Masters in 2007, I went to Pune for six months for some additional training, and then I joined Bhaktivedanta Hospital together with my wife, who is also an Ayurvedic doctor.

Ayurveda is the system of medicine that that treats people holistically, mostly using herbal remedies, and recommending lifestyle changes that incorporate practices like yoga, acupuncture, and massage. In Ayurveda we learn about how the body, mind, and soul are connected, and therefore one must constantly evaluate one's diet, level of exercise, sleep patterns, and stress management to be healthy. Ayurveda categorizes people into three *doshas*. *Doshas* are energies that circulate throughout the body, governing physical and mental processes. People in each dosha have certain emotional and physical commonalities, which have implications on the ideal lifestyle for each type. Most people are dominated by one or two *doshas*. The three *doshas* are: *Pita, Vata,* and *Kapha.*

According to Ayurveda, all of these types have to eat, behave, and be treated differently in order to maintain balance.

❦ ❦ ❦ ❦

Ayurveda and Spirituality

In medical school, I remember some of the professors would refer to the principles of *bhakti* and tell us that they wouldn't be useful for us in our careers. "What's the point of knowing about the soul, or about God?" they'd say. "This knowledge won't help you treat patients." I was really uncomfortable with this; I knew that spirituality meant a particular lifestyle that is exactly aligned with Ayurveda, and that this knowledge would be hugely beneficial to patients for both treatment and prevention of disease. That's why I was so attracted to the classes by the devotees, which were filled with practical, spiritual principles applicable to anyone. These classes, and those of Radhanath Swami, have deepened my understanding of Ayurveda. The main reason I accepted this opportunity at Bhaktivedanta Hospital was because I knew Ayurveda could be more effective if administered it in a spiritual environment.

❦ ❦ ❦ ❦

A Holistic Approach

Ayurveda is not a replacement for allopathic medicine. There is a place for both. For example, Ayurveda is excellent to treat some chronic or lifestyle-related conditions, for preventative care, and for mild or non-urgent conditions, among other things. Allopathic medicine is right for emergency or acute conditions, rapid symptom relief, and severe infections, among other things. There are also situations when an integrated approach is the right option, for example with some chronic conditions, rehabilitation, or stress and mental health. The key is to consult a physician, and here at the Bhaktivedanta Hospital, all doctors have a well-rounded, informed approach to care.

Ayurveda consists of medicinal plus lifestyle changes. We all must live a lifestyle in the mode of goodness—we must have healthy and wise habits. We must look after our mental, social, spiritual, and physical health. I stress this with all my patients.

When patients first arrive, we administer an Ayurvedic questionnaire that gives us a glimpse into the patient's lifestyle. From there, it's very easy to understand some of the causes of their diseases. For example, suppose someone has childhood asthma. In Mumbai, cases of childhood asthma have increased significantly over the last 10-15 years. One interesting thing we observed is that sometimes, the cause of asthma in children is the feeling of insecurity, or a lack of love. If parents aren't spending enough time with their kids, or if kids are not being fed properly, this reduces a child's mental capacity as well. In this way, the child becomes insecure and begins to be fearful. Fear negatively impacts one's respiratory tract. As per Ayurvedic understanding, desire, lamentation, and fear negatively affect the circulation of air in the body. It is said that all diseases, physical and mental, are caused by poor or inefficient circulation of air in the body. It may sound too simple, or even crazy, but showering children with love by giving them time and attention can actually reverse diseases like asthma—I've seen it myself. I recently dealt with a family with an asthmatic child. When we realized that the parents weren't spending enough time with the child due to work commitments, the mother decided to create an arrangement at work that allowed her to work from home, and therefore to spend a lot more quality time with her daughter. Within one month, the daughter's asthma completely went away.

Of course, I'm not suggesting that all asthma is caused by insecurity or lack of love; however, I have seen this to be the case many times.

The lifestyle questionnaire often reveals dietary habits that provide insight into causes of illnesses as well. One cannot underestimate the impact of food on the consciousness. People think that food only affects physical health, but it affects mental health as well.

We've helped families deal with depression, marital problems, parenting, and so much more, just with the principles of Ayurveda. One couple came to see me about curing a snoring problem. Due to the man's snoring, the couple, who had been married for 32 years, hadn't slept in the same bedroom for 30 years! The woman had said that this physical distance had caused an emotional distance in their marriage. After questioning them about their lifestyle, it was revealed that the couple would cook all the meals for the week every Saturday. Eating non-fresh, stored foods will decrease the fire of digestion, and that causes the mouth to stay open while one is asleep. This makes the tongue roll backwards, which, in turn, instigates snoring. When the couple began to eat fresh foods daily, the snoring went away.

I also coached a young man, about 22 years old, to better health by teaching him the importance of forgiveness. He was experiencing digestive issues that reduced significantly after we began practically applying the principles of forgiveness in his life.

In my experience, there are three ways to get mental

peace: the first is to sleep on time. The second is to have good relationships. And the third is to adopt spirituality. These three things, if tended to carefully, will allow you to deal with your issues peacefully; otherwise, small issues will provoke you. Spirituality and good relationships are strongly affected by good sleep. We need to sleep well, and enough, to be healthy and vibrant. In fact, Krishna even says in the *Bhagavad-gita* that one must be regulated in eating, sleeping, recreation, and work in order to mitigate the pangs of material life.

There's no doubt that Ayurveda has a place in a holistic care facility; it can aid in physical, mental, emotional, and social wellness. It has a very positive effect on society at large.

Interview with Shraboni Gupta

Spiritual Care Nurse
February 12, 2014

I used to feel shy to tell my story, because I was ashamed. But, I don't feel that way anymore. I've learned that sharing my story with others is healing for them, and for me, too. Still, I weep when I tell it.

I was born in Bandra to a wholesome family. My parents were in a happy marriage, and my siblings and I grew up feeling confident and grounded.

In 1998, when I was 19, my parents met a family with a 27-year-old son, and soon felt that he and I would be a good match. He is from the same caste, and shares my love of music. He is a classical singer, and actually, his whole family is very artistic. They are *tabla* players, *kattak* dancers, and singers. I have loved music my whole life; I even studied it in school. Singing especially, is my artistic passion.

Some of my friends were getting married around that time, so when our parents suggested we get married that year, I got caught up in the excitement of it all. My fiancé and I discovered all the ways we seemed to have so much in common—from music, to art, to dancing. We had a short but really lovely engagement.

From the second day of my marriage, though, I realized that this family wasn't who they said they were. They sometimes act kind outside of the house, but inside the house, they are terrible to each other. They argue, they slap each other and even others mid-conversation, and they are suspicious of everyone. They believe the worst in everyone. They create so many problems in their own minds. They were emotionally abusive to me, and to each other.

Very soon, my husband became physically violent with me. It was episodic, and unpredictable. I didn't tell my parents about the violent episodes, because I didn't want them to be worried. Soon, my parents could sense that I was acting differently. I wasn't as joyful, or as talkative. They asked me many times if I was okay, but I could never bring myself to tell them the truth.

When I looked into my husband's history, I saw that he was on medication for mental illness. He would tell me when he'd go to the doctor, but he never told me that actually, he was seeing a psychiatrist. I soon discovered that the entire family has a long and complex history of mental illness, that they didn't disclose before we got married.

I felt trapped, and tricked into marriage.

My parents always taught me, my whole life, that every marriage has its problems and that divorce is never an option. Indian culture values tolerance and the ability to adjust. Now, I understand that this doesn't mean to tolerate abuse. But I didn't get it then. In the name of tolerating and adjusting, it just never occurred to me to leave my husband—I just thought that every marriage was hard, and I had to stick it out and work through it. In those early days, my husband was either indifferent or violent—but never affectionate.

In 2000, we moved close to Mira Road and I started going to the Radha-Giridhari temple. I was always very spiritually inclined, so I was happy to see that there was a temple close to our new home. The devotees there really inspired me, and I began to feel the desire to serve others reawaken in me. In the midst of all my grief and suffering, I had lost myself. Coming in contact with this temple made me feel reacquainted with myself—with my desire to serve others, and my love of music. At the temple, I started singing and even leading *kirtan*, and it felt so therapeutic, to combine my love of music with spirituality. I really found peace in *kirtan*. I absolutely loved it. Slowly, I started to practice a little bit of *bhakti* at home as well. My husband would come with me to the temple sometimes, too.

In late 2001, I became pregnant. Upon hearing the news, my husband became ecstatic, and started treating me very well. He was no longer violent. It felt like he was really trying to be a good person, the best version of himself. I had a very healthy pregnancy. I was being treated here at Bhaktivedanta Hospital, and was well looked after. It felt like life was finally somewhat peaceful. In the ninth month, as is customary in India, I went to stay with my mother and I ended up giving birth at a hospital close to her house. Unfortunately, there were a lot of complications with the labour. There were junior doctors there who had no idea what to do with me. They shifted me to another hospital. I was so afraid. Finally, our beautiful daughter Sundari was born, in July of 2002. I was so happy, but in so much pain and extremely weak. From the hospital, I went back to my mother's house. Nine days later, my husband and in-laws asked me to come back home. So I did, even though I wanted to stay with my mom longer.

I had never seen my husband so happy. He would constantly play with Sundari, and take care of me. It was the best I'd ever seen him. He was kind, affectionate, and I actually felt protected.

Sadly, it was short lived. After just a couple of weeks, he became suspicious of me. Why? Because I had a male doctor. My husband was convinced that Sundari and I didn't need to see the doctor so often, and that there was something going on between him and me. I felt so emotionally battered, and my body was still recovering from childbirth.

My daughter had some health issues as well, so between managing her and my health issues, and cooking and doing all the housework, I was completely exhausted.

One day, out of nowhere, I blacked out and fell to the ground. I came to the Bhaktivedanta Hospital for treatment, and Dr. Dalal told me I had diminished blood in my body and needed transfusions.

Around the same time, my husband's health also took a turn for the worse, and he was frequently being admitted to the hospital for days at a time. I'd be looking after Sundari on my own or sending her to my mom's house for a few days. My husband stopped working regularly and we were suffering financially. Then he started smoking as well. He was only interacting with his mom and dad, who somehow didn't seem to worry about him. He became depressed. He lost all ability and desire to have discipline, or routine, and felt incapable of showing any interest or concern for me or Sundari. The medications he was prescribed seemed to exacerbate everything.

I started teaching and tutoring to help make ends meet. I never pursued a bachelor's degree because I married so young. But I was able to tutor and bring home some humble earnings. My brothers also supported us financially to the extent they could. After a little while, Sundari and I moved in with my mother. It made more sense—my mother was watching Sundari practically every day anyway. And, I just wanted Sundari to feel like she had a family. I was so confused and emotionally distraught. I was worried about my daughter in both homes—at my mom's house, I worried that she didn't have the love of her father. At my husband's house, I was worried that she was being exposed to too much negativity. I'm a very emotional person—it's proven to be both a blessing and a curse in my life. I thought,

"What did Sundari do wrong? Why does she have to deal with an absent father?" I was so angry! But almost immediately, I changed my mind, and moved back in with my husband. After everything, I still saw the good in him and was desperate for Sundari to have a regular family. I went back to my husband, and I begged him to please stop smoking, to take care of his health, and to be a better father.

And it worked. He started to change. He found the right medications for his mental health conditions, and started giving me and Sundari his time and attention again. He also returned to work, and started singing again.

I've been married now for 14 years. My child is almost 12 years old and taller than me. We're living as normal a life as we can. My husband is not violent anymore, and he's never, ever been abusive to our daughter. He gets angry and depressed easily, and he often lashes out at me. But, he is in therapy now, and I see him trying to take responsibility for his behaviour more than ever before.

You know, when he sings, I feel like he's the best singer in the entire world. He's got a beautiful voice. I beg Krishna to please let him use his talent for spiritual purposes, and to please give me strength to carry on. Mental illness is very complex. Before I understood what was happening with him, I honestly would have thoughts of taking my own life. But coming in contact with the Radha-Giridhari temple, and having my daughter, are the two things that saved me. I started chanting Hare Krishna regularly after Sundari was born, and I can see the difference it's made in my life. I feel calmer, wiser, and more at peace.

In 2011, I joined the Bhaktivedanta Hospital as a counsellor. Both Sundari and I had been patients at this hospital, and every time we came, we felt inspired, worthy, and so loved. We were surrounded by kindness. I was enjoying tutoring children, and I began doing it more regularly. But, I was missing something. I really wanted to serve more people, and I always had an interest in counselling. I had learned so much through my struggles in my marriage, and by being able to contextualize my suffering through *bhakti*, and I was eager to help others as well. So, I completed some training, applied, and was hired to be a member of the Spiritual Care Team.

Here at the hospital, I meet so many people, of all walks of life. I meet people of all races, nationalities, religions. I meet people in happy marriages, and in miserable marriages. I meet wealthy people, and I meet impoverished people. I meet people who suffer from very serious physical diseases or psychological trauma. I've realized that every single person in this world is suffering. Every single person struggles in the same ways even if it may present differently—we really are one human race. Whether one is a Hare Krishna or a Muslim or a Christian or a Jew—we are all the same. Krishna loves all of us. It really doesn't matter what name we give God, we are all brothers and sisters. This has been my strongest realization working here. It's also put my own suffering into perspective—we all suffer. I can draw from my suffering to help others, and for this, I'm deeply grateful. My suffering has genuinely made me a better counsellor. I've been able to help so many people, just like I've been helped. I've also realized very clearly that I'm just a medium, an instrument. Prabhupada has given me the ability and opportunity to help, and because of that, I see miracles every day.

☙ ☙ ☙

Hospital Inspiration

I remember one patient, a 42-year-old woman named Priya, who is a devout Buddhist. She was hospitalized in the middle of January 2012 due to an abdominal wound that required an operation. She was in a lot of pain. I went to meet with her and collected her lifestyle information. After some time, she began to trust me and we developed a nice friendship. She would tell me for hours about her life, her fears, her belief in God. She said that this hospital made her feel closer to Lord Buddha. I encouraged her in her spiritual practice. She was afraid about her upcoming operation, and I asked her how I could help to alleviate her fear. She asked me to read to her from the *Bhagavad-gita As It Is*. She said it made her feel peaceful. I told her to pray, and we both meditated together. When she was being wheeled into the Operation Theatre and then later into the recovery room, she held my hand very tight. While she was in recovery, she asked me to chant a prayer of protection for her. I sang the *Nrisimhadeva* Prayers and we again prayed and meditated together. She was here for 20 days because she needed to be kept for observation. I would go to her every day, and we'd read together. She told me more about her guru and her spiritual practice. It was so interesting. I told her that we are all spiritual beings and it is our true nature to live clean, happy, spiritual lives. She had a lot of faith in her spiritual practice and that made me very happy.

She said, "Your *Bhagavad-gita* is universally applicable—please keep reading it to me."

So I did. I told her she's right; the philosophy espoused in the *Bhagavad-gita As It Is* is non-sectarian, and can be followed by anyone regardless of what aspect of God they believe in. It's a philosophy for the soul, regardless of the type of body it's in. It is accepted everywhere around the world. She actually ended up getting one for herself.

Priya had a 10-year-old daughter at the time, whose birthday was coming up. Unfortunately, she wouldn't be well enough to go home to celebrate, and this really upset her daughter. Priya told her, "Don't worry, I'll be celebrating your birthday here!" When we heard this, the staff threw a party for the little girl. I gifted her with a colouring book and a storybook, and I arranged for a cake. The staff and volunteers here that day poured affection and blessings on her. Priya was so happy—she said it was better than anything she could have planned herself at home.

Priya is now healthy and thriving. She can't come to programs at the hospital very often because she lives quite far away, but we are in touch almost every day. Whenever she can, she comes to visit me. She also sends her relatives here for treatment whenever required. She told me that she felt completely comfortable to follow her own religious beliefs while staying at this hospital, and that she left feeling more spiritually inspired.

Another person I always remember is a Muslim woman named Reshma, whose mother was admitted here. Her mother was Hindu, and Reshma was Hindu and had converted to Islam after getting married. She asked me if I could read to her mother from the *Bhagavad-gita As It Is*. She said, "My sister and I both married into Muslim families and have converted to Islam. Now we know about both religions, and we've realized that, actually, God is one." I've never come across a Muslim patient who objected to the prayers we sing for them or for other patients. They always say, "Allah is one, and we can all pray."

Reshma said she and her family were so happy to be in a hospital that was so clean, and where they could easily do their daily *namaz* prayers and be encouraged to do them. They grew very attached to their doctors, and whenever any of them have a health issue, they return here.

Somehow, while being with this family it occurred to me

that Srila Prabhupada had called them here. They were his guests. Somehow or other, people come here to this hospital, at Srila Prabhupada's home, to get treatment for their bodies, minds, and souls. For us to actually do that effectively, we have to be instruments of Srila Prabhupada's compassion. That is all we are—instruments. Vehicles for Srila Prabhupada to use to transmit his care and attention to the people he calls here. I want that whoever comes here leaves feeling closer to God—however he manifests for them, whatever they call him. I pray that everyone always leaves with a good impression of this hospital and of Srila Prabhupada.

Every day I pray for more determination to serve better. I know it's not in my power to help others; I'm being empowered and, in the process, it's helping me too. I feel protected here.

Sundari also likes to come to the hospital and play with the younger patients. Just the other day, she was playing with a young patient her age, and they were practicing dance moves together! She is becoming such a wonderful *katthak* dancer. My wish is that she will dance in front of the Jagannath deity, and sing classical music in Vrindavan. This morning, we were singing the prayer *Nitai Pada Kamala* in a Bengali tune, she was dancing along. The way she dances is simply amazing. I will sing for you now—*Nitai Pada Kamala*. Oh, you should hear the tunes my husband sings; they're so sweet.

I think everyone deserves love, even people who are hurtful towards others. Everyone needs appreciation. At the courses here in the hospital, I've learned a lot about compassionate communication that I apply at home and at work. Empathic listening, reflective listening, self-appreciation. If we think positively, we attract positivity. I've also learned a lot about forgiveness. Until we forgive with our hearts, how will Krishna reveal himself?

The tears in my eyes right now are tears of happiness. Krishna is so kind to give me my pain because it's made me better, stronger, wiser. I can feel his love and care for me. I know I wouldn't be able to perceive it as much if everything in my life was perfect. So while I'd never want to relive those darker days, I can only be grateful for them, because they led me to this faith, and this job, which has given me true purpose and meaning. What else could I ask for?

Interview with Priyanka Agarwal

Patient & Patient Family Member
January 31, 2014

Finding Bhaktivedanta Hospital

I have been sick a lot in my life. I have been treated at so many hospitals that I've lost count. I came upon the Bhaktivedanta Hospital years ago, when there was a natural disaster in Gujarat. Some patients from Gujarat were transferred to Mumbai and were treated here at Bhaktivedanta Hospital. I was deeply emotional about the catastrophe, and I wanted to help. When I found out patients from Gujarat were being treated here, I called to see if I can bring food and clothing for the patients, as I don't live too far from Mira Road. That was how I first became acquainted with this hospital.

I expected panic. Horrible smells. The sounds of depression.

But I experienced none of that here. In the midst of this tragedy, why was I finding myself in an atmosphere of... joy?

✤ ✤ ✤ ✤

Becoming a Patient, and a Patient Family Member

After that experience, I started coming here for all of my health struggles. The first time I was admitted here, it was because I needed dialysis. Then, in 2000, I was admitted several times because I contracted tuberculosis. Then there were problems with my diabetes, and I even had an angina attack and was admitted in the ICU.

While all this was happening, my dad was also continuously getting sick. A sonography report revealed he could have lung cancer, and Dr. Dhaval Dalal referred us to a specialist in Kandivali. That specialist later confirmed that it was indeed lung cancer. In January 2008, my dad got really sick. I was still in close contact with Dr. Dalal because of my own maladies, and I'd always talk to him about what was happening with my father. Dr. Dalal is also like my father—as well as being like my brother and friend. In fact, I feel that I'm here today, able to speak to you, only because of him. In his treatment there is so much love and prayer. He advised me to purchase an oxygen tank for my dad, as it would be required at home. But after just a few days of using it, my father still couldn't breathe properly, and he even stopped eating and drinking. I was so scared. I told Dr. Dalal, and he told me to bring my dad here immediately, to the ICU.

When we arrived, the doctors told me my father was in the process of dying. Naturally overwhelmed, I just fell in front of the deity of Srila Prabhupada. While I don't consider myself a *bhakti* practitioner, I believe Srila Prabhupada is an incredible man of God, and at that moment, I felt completely broken and I wanted to talk to him. I felt like I was losing consciousness. I prayed for the strength to get through this. The doctors, my sister, my brother-in-law, and my then husband all came and tried to comfort me, but it was so overwhelming.

I never talked to my dad about his cancer. Dr. Dalal kept telling me I should, but I felt that he was so weak that he wouldn't have been able to handle the negativity. I just kept lying to him and telling him he'd be okay, hoping that a positive attitude would help make him better.

Once I understood that he was dying, I began to think of how to make his departure as dignified and painless as possible. He had recently become a *bhakti* practitioner. He often went to the Radha-Rasabihari temple. I knew he'd want to die in the ideal way for a *bhakti-yogi*. I asked the doctor, "How can I arrange a *tulasi* leaf and some *ganga jal* for my dad?"

"Don't worry, I'll arrange it," he said. I can't explain how grateful I felt at that moment.

One day, I was sitting outside the ICU, and one of the Spiritual Care nurses, Gaurangi, approached me with a smile. "How are you doing?" she asked gently, putting a hand on my shoulder. "Is there anything I can do for you?"

"I'm not sure," I said. "Maybe we could pray and read *Bhagavad-gita* together? My father has always encouraged me to read it."

"Of course," she said.

My whole life, I never really felt connected to Krishna. I believe in God, but I never really thought of Krishna as the supreme God, and I definitely never felt like I had a relationship with him.

But that day with Gaurangi, I started to read the *Bhagavad-gita As It Is*, which is a conversation between Krishna and his friend Arjun. After that, I used to come daily at 5 p.m. to visit my dad, and Gaurangi would meet me and take me to my father's room. Together, we would read and discuss the *Gita*. She would read me a Sanskrit verse, then we would discuss it, and sing Hare Krishna. After some time, I could feel Krishna making his way into a tiny corner of my heart.

I started to sing Hare Krishna at home on my own. I'd catch myself doing it again and again.

I'm not a big devotee like everyone here, but I did start to feel closer to Krishna after a little while. I started talking to him all the time. My dad gave me a picture of Krishna, and I would regularly make cup of tea, sit before this picture, and talk to him. I still do that now. Soon, I felt inspired to change my eating habits to align with what the *Gita* suggests in order to have a healthy and spiritual life.

One day, in February of 2008, I had a horrible feeling of panic. I knew something was wrong. I called Gaurangi and asked her if she could meet me earlier than we had planned, and if she could take me to see my dad. I just didn't want to wait. She said yes, and I went to the hospital, whereupon she immediately took me to the ICU. I just had to see my father.

I had brought some Radha-Giridhari *prasadam* with me and gave it to my father along with some *ganga jal* and *tulasi*. Then, Gaurangi and I went outside his room and started reading together. All of a sudden, at about 6:30 p.m., Dr. Dalal hurried into the room, and I saw him make a cross on his paper. I froze; I knew what that meant. It was an indication that they were no longer to administer any medication, because his body was simply shutting down. I went into my father's room and held his hand. He was smiling at me. I told him not to worry.

At 9:45 p.m., I was holding my dad's hand with my right hand, my *Bhagavad-gita* in my left, and reading to him while he was looking at a picture of Krishna. As I was reading, my husband, brother, and others were coming in and checking on us, looking at the monitors. I was about to finish a verse, when I noticed that my dad was no more. My husband came in and said, "Priyanka, he's gone."

"Don't disturb me," I said. "I need to finish reading this verse to him."

I finished the verse, chanted a little, and closed daddy's eyes. I could see from all the monitors that he was no longer in his body. At that moment, there was not one drop of water in my eyes—I felt this strength that Gaurangi equipped me with, and the knowledge that while this journey may be very much over, daddy was still very much alive, just no longer in this body. And as his daughter, I felt relieved that I was able to send him off in the way he wanted—hearing about his Krishna. I felt like I did what I came to do.

My brother was hysterical, and I had to calm him down. I told him, "He just left his dress—this body was just a dress for him, the soul. I don't know what dress God will give him now, but I know he'll be okay. Please, let him go peacefully."

I cry every time I think about that moment. I'm his younger sister. We wiped our tears, and took him to the morgue.

After my dad died, my health continued to deteriorate. I had serious diabetic attacks, and later experienced a lot of uterine bleeding. A doctor here performed uterine fibroid embolization, and then in August 2011, I had a hysterectomy. And after that, I also had cataract surgery. My body is a disaster. But my spirit thrives.

Interview with Radhanath Swami

Spiritual Teacher and Guide for
Bhaktivedanta Hospital Founding Doctors and
New York Times Bestselling Author
Summer 2019, New York City

I was born in Chicago in 1950. During the '50s and '60s there was a growing conflict in my mind. The world seemed to be filled with negativity. There was widespread racism, arrogance, and hate, sometimes even in the name of religion. Happiness seemed superficial to me in the face of people suffering prejudice and injustice due to their race or religion. At that time, the Vietnam war was raging. The war didn't really make sense to many of us. I became a serious activist in the civil rights movement and the counterculture. Gradually, though, I realized that to help bring real, substantial change to the world, there needed to be a spiritual transformation in people's hearts. So I embarked upon a spiritual search, a journey of self-discovery.

I hitchhiked from London through Europe and the Middle East, to India. I aspired to experience the values and lifestyles of people in other countries. I was especially fascinated with studying various conceptions of God and how those conceptions could define our interactions with each other and with nature.

After travelling overland for six months, I finally arrived at the border of India. It was December of 1970. There, I was rejected entry because I had only $0.26, and I was told that I required a minimum of $200 to enter. I begged and begged to no avail. Angered by my persistence, immigration and assembled military guards screamed, "Go back to where you came from, we have enough beggars in India!"

The immigration 'office' in that place was a single desk under some trees in a field flanked with a foreboding metal fence topped with swirling barbed wire. I withdrew back into the no-man's land between India and Pakistan from where I had come. There, I sat under a tree and helplessly prayed. After a several hours, the immigration guards completed their shift, and new agents arrived to begin theirs. I approached a new immigration agent and pleaded, "I have hitchhiked across the whole world to meet your people and understand your culture. I promise you, if you just give me a chance, someday I'll do something good for the people of India."

The guard was a Sikh gentleman, maybe 60 years old. I was 19. After an intense, prolonged stare into my eyes, he spoke, "My commanding officer ordered me to reject you, but sometimes a man must follow his heart. I will give you the chance that you are crying for." Then, he put his hand on my head and said, "Son, may God bless you with what you're longing to receive. Welcome to India." With that, he stamped my passport.[8]

The greatest treasures of my life, I received in India. I still feel so indebted. I wandered all around India and studied various forms of Buddhism, Hinduism, Islam, Christianity, and Baha'i. I strived to deeply experience whatever I was learning and practicing.

Ultimately, I was led to the holy place of Vrindavan and discovered the path of devotion to Krishna. I found this to be the fulfillment of all my prayers. In Vrindavan, I aspired to give my life to the beautiful path of *bhakti*. It was there that I met my guru, A.C. Bhaktivedanta Swami Prabhupada, and offered my heart to serve him. Eventually

---

8. Those who are interested can read the Swami's full autobiography in his book entitled *The Journey Home*, and its sequel, *The Journey Within*.

my visa expired and I had to depart from India. At that time, I came back to the West and became a part of the Krishna Consciousness society.

In the West, for some time, I was stationed in the Appalachian mountains. I was taking care of cows in an old barn, and deities on an altar in a farm house. I was very happy there, though I was always missing Vrindavan. Then, beginning in 1979, my life was devoted to sharing *bhakti* by travelling to universities, colleges, and communities in the mid-eastern area of the United States.

Eventually, in 1987, destiny brought me back to India. In South Mumbai, each day I was offering programs in people's homes and lecturing in colleges and universities. That's when something very special started to happen in Mumbai. A congregation was growing. Over time, a wonderful, thriving community of devotees formed in the Chowpatty area of South Mumbai.

There were a few young men in the congregation who were medical school students: Ajay, Girish, Vivek, and Dhaval. Only Vivek was married. The others, being unmarried, wanted to leave school to join the *ashram* and become renounced monks. I encouraged them to complete their medical degrees. Once their degrees were completed, they were encouraged to receive specialty degrees.

After graduation, the medical students all married incredibly intelligent and devoted partners, some of whom were also doctors. They found a collective purpose in sharing pure love of God while practicing holistic medical care. They were devoted to integrating genuine spirituality with their particular branches of medical practice.

We encouraged them, as a group, to serve *together* and create something wonderful. We had a vision of what these young doctors could accomplish. It was like a seed; we really didn't know how that seed would grow, but we had faith that it would.

At one point, we all decided that we should open a full-scale hospital. Hrishikesh Mafatlal, a truly compassionate businessman, was the most excited of all—and that was the beginning of the Bhaktivedanta Hospital. From that time, we became an intimate, dedicated family and a united team.

Ram Maheshwar and Hrishikesh procured an excellent plot of land in Mira Road. A devoted team including Dr. Bimal Shah began designing the building. We wanted the hospital to mirror the temple project in Mayapur, with similar colours and architectural designs. Srila Prabhupada led the design of the first buildings in the Mayapur Hare Krishna campus, and we tried to bring that spirit into the hospital.

Because the hospital was being named after His Divine Grace A. C. Bhaktivedanta Swami Prabhupada, our team strived to develop every aspect of the hospital with excellence and precision, just as Srila Prabhupada did with everything he created. From the beginning, the goal was to create a hospital dedicated to the body, mind, and soul. There are so many hospitals for the body, some for the mind, but not many that aim to genuinely awaken souls to their higher spiritual potential. Compassion for the body and mind is urgently required, yet the highest compassion and the most pressing need is to awaken the soul. This spiritual awakening is the most comprehensive solution for suffering. With this aspiration, the Spiritual Care department was formed. It is the very heart of the hospital.

The early days were difficult; running a hospital proved to be very challenging. There were so many urgent demands. One day, I visited the hospital and I asked about the Spiritual Care department. They told me that it hardly existed anymore. It was still a department, but barely anything was happening due to the demanding needs of running a hospital.

So, in an affectionate, but strong way, I presented to them the primary purpose of the hospital – to provide spiritual care. Unless we made it a top priority, it would never manifest. I stressed to the doctors, "All the things you're doing are tangible, necessary, and demanding. But in order for spiritual care to exist, we have to establish it as our top priority; everything else has to revolve around it—otherwise, it will be forgotten." Sometimes we place higher importance on those things that produce tangible results relatively quickly. For example, after an hour of work, you might get a tangible result, be it financial, or maybe experiential. But it's often the activities that don't produce a tangible result immediately, that are of utmost value. We tend to measure success by quantitative metrics rather than by the quality of our character and purpose. It's similar to our spiritual practice—it doesn't always produce a tangible result that we can see. Still, we understand that our spiritual practice, our *sadhana*, is at the heart of connecting us to God and to ourselves.

At the time, Ajay was the Director of the hospital. Soon after our conversation, he humbly stepped down from his position and volunteered to lead the Spiritual Care team. No one asked him to do it, but he knew what had to be done. And he did it for several years. Ajay took the lead with great support from Vivek, and they created the Spiritual Care team as systematically and scientifically as any medical science. They created a structure with the same precision and sense of care as running the Operating Room! They took great responsibility to design a system and train qualified practitioners. Their aim was to inspire and implement a non-sectarian Spiritual Care department that would inspire people of all faiths. There are Muslim, Christian, Sikh, Jewish, Jain, Parsi, and Hindu patients, so the spiritual care had to be relevant to all. We strive to base our spiritual care on universal principles without compromising the essence of spirituality. Ajay put his heart and soul into building the whole team, and because he was the Director of the hospital and highly respected, everyone understood that what he was doing was of utmost importance. Prior to this, the medical staff took each other very seriously, but the Spiritual Care team wasn't taken as seriously; it was just a program that was part of it all, but it was neglected. When Ajay took charge of the department, it gave a signal to everyone that this department was at the heart of everything we were doing. Spiritual care became core to the identity of the Bhaktivedanta Hospital.

Spiritual care was not limited to only the patients; it was also provided for the relatives of the patients, the hospital staff, and the entire community surrounding the hospital. It eventually became so effective that other hospitals began contacting us to help them implement spiritual care in their institutions. Patients didn't feel pressured or preached to. Rather, the consistent feedback received was that they felt they were being enlightened and cared for in a spiritual environment.

Another way we focused on spiritual care was to be more intentional about honouring the hospital's name. As mentioned, it was named after His Divine Grace A.C. Bhaktivedanta Swami Prabhupada. We were careful to put Srila Prabhupada's service in the centre by the way we nourished a culture of devotional service. We placed Srila Prabhupada's deity in the centre of the main entrance lobby. Three times a day, staff members who were so inclined participated in prayer by gathering around Srila Prabhupada and reciting the beautiful Sanskrit verses known as Siksastakam, followed by a brief talk by one of the senior staff members.

The hospital community became very spiritually focused. It felt like everything was running more smoothly.

🙏 🙏 🙏 🙏

Troubling Times

Then came a great crisis. A powerful political party sought control over the hospital, claiming that we were underpaying several staff members. In truth, we were doing our best – balancing limited resources to offer both fair compensation and affordable healthcare. Despite our efforts to reach a mutual understanding, tensions escalated.

What followed was intense and painful. The hospital came under attack—windows were broken, staff members were assaulted and even harassed at their homes. For some of our team, essential utilities like electricity and water were cut off. The oppression became so severe that we had no choice but to close the hospital.

The hospital remained closed for a year. It was extremely intense; the founders were thinking of relocating, and starting another hospital in a friendlier area.

We committed ourselves to remain in the same location, but we had to sincerely re-evaluate our original purpose. We had already refocused on Spiritual Care, and we became more adept at the business side of running a hospital, but we had to re-stress our desire to be a missionary hospital that would provide for all—staff, patients, everyone—regardless of their means. We realized we needed to increase some salaries while continuing to keep patient costs low, all without falling into debt.

We created a fundraising department. Not just to subsidize the healthcare we were providing, but also to subsidize the salaries of a stratum of our staff members. It was a bold move; few hospitals need to raise funds to increase staff salaries.

After one year, we re-opened the hospital. Nobody really knew what was going to happen. Yet within a year of reopening, our income doubled. Today, it's nearly 20 times what it once was. It was a powerful confirmation that when Krishna is pleased, he empowers our efforts in extraordinary ways.

The fundraising department now supports a wide range of initiatives including hospital expansion, advanced medical equipment, and the opening of new branches. But one principle remains at the core: the spirit of compassion must guide all decisions. Everything else is secondary.

Looking back, the labour strike was, in truth, Krishna's grace. It humbled us, refocused us, and ultimately strengthened the very foundation of who we are.

We also rebuilt trust—within our team, with our patients, and across the wider community. Even the party that once opposed us came to respect our ethos, and some became advocates and allies.

Our purpose has always been not just to make profits, but to transform hearts. People's hearts will be changed if they see that our professional and business practices are dedicated to earnestly caring for them.

Along with the growing popularity of the hospital, spiritual care continued to thrive. It is interesting how when devotees implement their own practices of love for God in a kind, respectful, and non-judgemental way, people open their hearts to appreciate it; even if it may be foreign to their own background. For example, each day, nurses bring the deity of Jagannath to each patient's room on a rolling cart, like a miniature *Ratha Yatra*[9] festival! People of all faiths are offering flowers and taking *caranamrita*, illustrating that when worship is done with affection, without being judgemental, then it is truly non-sectarian. All sorts of people love to participate in this simple tradition because they see and feel that we are not trying to impose our beliefs on them—rather, we are sharing beautiful ways of celebrating *bhakti*, which espouses love for all living entities, regardless of religion, caste, or creed. Srila Prabhupada said at times that our success is to help Christians become better Christians, Jews better Jews, Muslims better Muslims, and so on. Countless people leave from the hospital feeling their lives enriched, more peaceful, and more deeply connected to the God of their own faith.

And, it is wonderful to see how several thousand people have become *bhakti* practitioners and have formally accepted gurus within the *bhakti* tradition as a result of their association with Bhaktivedanta Hospital. It is all happening without any element of sectarian canvassing; people's hearts transform simply by associating with exemplary and kind devotees.

Even people considering themselves atheists often express appreciation for their experience at the hospital. They're personally treated with kindness, respect, and concern by doctors and nurses striving to selflessly serve. Association with sincere devotees is a powerful medicine that can heal the body, mind and soul.

A reason many people choose not to believe in God is that they see arrogance, division, and fighting among peo-

---

9. A chariot festival that originated in Jagannath Puri, India, wherein the deity is taken on a chariot on a parade. This festival now takes place around the world.

ple who do believe in God. This is a sad reality, though it's not how it is meant to be. The *Gita*, the Bible, the Quran, and all other genuine scriptures teach us that the origin of everything and everyone is God. To know, follow, and love God is the only true goal of life. For example, all music has its origin in glorifying or calling out for God's grace. The origin of most architecture was for the glory of God. The origin of many universities—Harvard, Princeton, Yale—all these universities were originally spiritual offerings. Of course, they later became influenced to be more professional and secular, but the origin was an offering to God. Even the old hospitals in the West—St. Francis, St. Jude—began as the result of religious denominations who wanted to serve humanity on behalf of God.

As time passed, music became more mundane, hospitals became more materialistic, and so on. But the origin in such spiritually-founded organizations was never only about making money; the money-making was primarily to sustain the spirit of compassion. However, in time, and in many cases, money became the central purpose, and compassion became secondary.

※ ※ ※ ※

Compassion and Community

The Bhaktivedanta Hospital strives to keep compassion and community at the forefront. We hope and pray that this spirit will be sustained in future generations. For this purpose the hospital leadership is endeavouring to establish policies, cultural norms, and responsible succession.

Everyone is in need of love and compassion. As a traveling monk, people are always approaching me with joys, heartbreaks, and crises. It is a very real and personal experience for me to feel how much the world is filled with suffering. There are so many reasons people suffer. For example, people suffer from a sense of meaninglessness, hopelessness, disconnection, and not knowing their purpose in life. Relationships feel empty, superficial. There is widespread betrayal, disappointment, and unmet expectations. Influenced by others, people develop extremely unrealistic expectations of their own selves. And they feel worthless, useless, and never good enough.

To deal with the various stresses, disappointments, and frustrations in life, millions of good-hearted people resort to intoxication and dangerous habits for an illusory sense of relief. And, there are people who instinctively hide from their vulnerabilities by developing hardened, arrogant, and unkind hearts. It's so common.

On top of all of that, we live in a world where vulnerability is often viewed as a weakness. This leads to people being afraid to openly share what they're going through. Or, they simply don't know how to share.

Emotional distress, especially when unexpressed, affects the body, and bodily distress affects the mind. Mental misery is sometimes more painful than physical misery. When patients talk about their problems, they need a loving ear, a friend to talk to. They need to know they're speaking with someone who genuinely cares.

Clearly, a person's physical well-being is just one aspect of their wellness. So many people die by suicide due to hopelessness while still having healthy bodies. This heartbreaking fate is often induced by depression, mental anguish, and a perceived lack of meaning.

The root of all these anomalies is a disconnection from one's original spiritual consciousness – forgetfulness of the innate love and joy of the soul that is transcendental to the ever-changing temporary world around us.

Actual healthcare has to be holistic; it needs to be for the body, mind, and soul. This is compassion.

Community, in Sanskrit, is called *Varnashram dharma*. At its core, this principle ensures that people from all walks of life are serving a common goal together, according to their interests, abilities, and natural inclinations, while simultaneously making spiritual progress.

To have a hospital, we need software engineers, plumbers, housekeepers, nurses, doctors, cooks, accountants, pharmacists, salespeople, business people, marketers, and more. We have an opportunity to bring all these people together to serve in a spiritual environment, while hearing spiritual sound vibrations and spreading love of God!

Our hospital offers many people the opportunity to be engaged and support their families in the setting of a spiritual community. Children who have grown up in the congregation, who have graduated from our schools, and children from our orphanage in Chowpatty, have chosen to engage in a devotional livelihood at Bhaktivedanta Hospital. Some are now heads of departments! Several of our monks, who have decided to change *ashram* and be married, have preferred to earn a livelihood in a spiritual atmosphere, and are employed at Bhaktivedanta Hospital. This is an important aspect of the hospital; to create a sort of *Varnashram* model where all kinds of people could find community and service amongst like-minded people and feel valued for who they are.

Another way we stress community, and one of the unique features of Bhaktivedanta Hospital, is that it incorporates several schools of medicine in one building, and the particular doctors of each school of medicine respect and harmonize with each other. You see, medicine is often like sectarian religion. In the sectarian fundamentalist version of any religion, there is a belief that their way is the only way, and all others are misled or evil. Medicine can be like that, too. There are some allopathic doctors who believe the traditions of natural medicine are influenced by witch doctors, superstition, and primitive practices. Then there are some natural medical traditions that see allopathy as poisoning people with deadly chemicals. I know Ayurvedic doctors that won't train allopathic doctors because they're already "ruined."

We have seen from Srila Prabhupada and his predecessor teachers, that all true religions can lead one to progressive levels of love for the One God. We respect and honour that. In a similar way, in relation to medical traditions, we've seen people get cured through the methods of naturopathy, homeopathy, yoga therapy and allopathy—each has its own special benefits. If a person comes into the Emergency Room after an accident and his insides are coming out, you can't treat him with homeopathic tablets! He will need surgery to save his life. It is common in Bhaktivedanta Hospital, with the patient's consent, to have a professional acupuncturist effectively administer acupuncture to people in pain while undergoing other treatments after surgeries. Ayurveda is excellent for overall health, treatment of disease, and preventative measures. *Panca-karma*[10] is a method proven over the centuries to cleanse and rejuvenate the body. In addition, after surgery or chemotherapy an Ayurvedic regimen can significantly restore a person's health. Bhaktivedanta Hospital has wings for Ayurveda, homeopathy, naturopathy, yoga therapy, acupuncture, psychology, and most branches of allopathy. They all serve together and appre-

---

10. An Ayurvedic detox process that gently cleanses the body of toxins. It involves five main therapies like oil massages, herbal enemas, and cleansing treatments. It is meant to restore balance in the body and mind.

ciate what each alternate branch can do. In our Integral Medicine department, doctors from all of these departments come together to discuss the best possible treatment for a particular patient.

Bhaktivedanta Hospital is also a research centre — they're doing research on addiction, sound therapy, *mantras*, near death experiences, and more. Our Govardhana Ecovillage[11], just outside of Mumbai, is also very closely connected to the hospital, so the whole idea of environmental, ecological, harmonious living is also being incorporated into the hospital. Bhaktivedanta Hospital is presently building a 100-bed missionary hospital at Govardhan Eco-village. It will be the only high-level hospital in the area of hundreds of simple villages.

It is a challenge is to preserve this vision. We know from experience that our ideals will inevitably be subject to diversion; that is the nature of the world. We need to sincerely embrace our ideals while regularly re-emphasizing our core purpose. With the grace of Krishna we pray that this service to God and humanity will be an offering that pleases the Lord.

※ ※ ※ ※

Nourishing the Soul

Some spiritual practitioners have criticized the hospital, saying it is focused on bodily welfare as opposed to providing eternal benefit.

More important than how we respond, is what we believe.

"*Bhakti*" means to engage in "devotional service," or service to the Lord with love. There are nine processes of

---

11. A beautiful retreat centre outside of Mumbai, based on the principles of *bhakti-yoga*.

devotional service to the Lord. It begins with associating with devotees, then hearing about the Lord, chanting sacred *mantras*, remembering the Lord, offering him personal service, praying, worshipping, befriending the Lord, and surrendering for the pleasure of the Lord. By following this process sincerely, we become rid of selfishness and egoism, and free from the modes of material nature. And at last, our natural love of God awakens.

There are three modes of material nature: goodness, passion, and ignorance. Our activities, thoughts, the food we eat, the music we listen to—everything can be categorized by these modes. The scriptures teach us how to elevate our consciousness to the mode of goodness and then, from the mode of goodness, to transcend the material modes and realize our true identity as a spirit soul who has a loving relationship with God. The path of *bhakti* gives all beings the opportunity to transcend the modes of material nature by practicing devotional service.

Srila Prabhupada described that opening hospitals is an activity in the mode of goodness. It is beneficial, of course, but in itself is limited to material philanthropy as it does not transcend the modes of nature; it does not nourish the soul, which is our true identity.

That said, this description by Srila Prabhupada does not apply to Bhaktivedanta Hospital, whose core goal and purpose is devotional service. Srila Prabhupada instructed us to engage our natures in the service of God. A well-known example is Srila Prabhupada encouraging George Harrison of the Beatles to dovetail his natural talent as a musician to share Krishna Consciousness with the world. This made Prabhupada so very happy.

Sri Caitanya Mahaprabhu, the most recent incarnation of Krishna who descended 500 years ago, gave a simple instruction to everyone: to dovetail one's occupational, social, and spiritual position in God's service while also sharing pure love of God.

The very purpose of Bhaktivedanta Hospital is to fulfill Srila Prabhupada's instructions by offering to him a united, like-minded community of responsible householders who earn their livelihood while inspiring love of God through devotional service according Lord Caitanya's teachings.

I have no adequate words to express my profound gratitude for each member of the community at Bhaktivedanta Hospital. I place my head and my heart at their feet with indebtedness. Their tireless efforts have attracted a shower of the Lord's grace to transform a hospital for those who are suffering, into a beautiful temple celebrating God's love.

Journal Entry: Meeting Madhava
Radha Bhakti
January 29, 2014

I arrive in my room at the hospital, exhausted after a day of intense interviews and meetings. I collapse on my bed, close my eyes, and exhale. Not even a second later, someone knocks on my door. I hastily get up, pull the latch to unlock the door and see Aleya, one of the Spiritual Care nurses.

"Madhava, you should meet him," she says. "But you must come right now!"

"Right, okay," I say, feeling frazzled.

I quickly grab my Dictaphone, bag, and keys, and hurriedly follow Aleya down a flight of stairs, left into a corridor, and into the first patient room on the right. I'm rather disoriented, and it occurs to me that I probably look exhausted and dishevelled. My mind is racing, but as soon as the door opens to the room, the noise in my head is silenced by the soft *beep beep beep* coming from a machine that I imagine is monitoring the patient's heartbeat, and the sound of Srila Prabhupada's voice faintly but clearly chanting the Hare Krishna *maha-mantra* from a small speaker beside the patient's bed.

Madhava, a terminal lung cancer patient, is sitting beside his bed in a chair. He is breathing with the help of tubes. His mother is sitting on the bench to his right, along with a nurse. His father is sitting on the bed, facing me, but not looking at me. He is looking down, on the floor. The mood is somber, juxtaposed by the big, beautiful rays of sunshine lighting up the room through the large windows on the wall facing me. Madhava greets me with a wonderful smile, so lovely that it actually takes me aback for a second.

"*Haribol!*" he says, as he gestures for me to sit on the bench next to him. His mother moves to the bed as she politely gives me a strained smile, barely making eye contact. Her pain is visible.

Between every couple of barely audible words, Madhava takes short, intentional breaths. It's a struggle for him to speak, and I feel guilty being here.

Should I really be bothering him? I think.

Madhava is gracious, and insists he is willing, and eager, to speak to me.

"My name is Radha," I say. "I'm visiting from Canada. I'm here interviewing staff and patients so I can write down their stories into what I hope will be a book."

"I see," he says with a smile and a nod.

"I'm hearing so many poignant stories about how people have been positively affected by the hospital. Thank you so much for letting me speak to you," I say.

"Not at all."

"Can you tell me a little bit about yourself?" I ask, feeling sheepish.

"I am a disciple of Murali Krishna Swami, whose guru is Gaur Govinda Swami, who was a disciple of Srila Prabhupada. My journey into *bhakti* was a fast one; I was completely taken by the philosophy as soon as I learned the golden lessons contained in the books of Srila Prabhupada. After I completed my studies, I immediately became a *bhakti* practitioner without wasting time. At first, my parents didn't really understand, but they came around."

"How old are you, *Prabhu?*" I ask.

"I am 29 years old," he says.

"*Prabhu,* why are you here at Bhaktivedanta Hospital?" I ask gently.

"I have lung cancer," he says. His eyes immediately start to water, and there is a long pause. Large tears fall from his face. He looks down, and quietly composes himself.

My eyes start to water, but I'm careful to ensure he doesn't notice. At this moment, there is nowhere else I want to be, but in this room with Madhava, to hear whatever he wants to share. I long to put my hand on his hand, but I am cognizant of the conservative culture in the hospital.

"I was living in Bhubaneswar and I was a regular member of the local temple congregation when I started feeling some pain in my back," he continues. "I went to the hospital and they said it was just a muscle spasm; nothing serious. So I left, but the pain was getting worse. I went to Rajasthan, to two or three hospitals, and everyone said that everything was okay. My MRI, blood tests, CT scans—everything was perfect. I came to Mumbai to visit a friend, and he insisted I get checked out here at the Bhaktivedanta Hospital. Then, all of a sudden, it was revealed that I was in the final stages of lung cancer."

Final stages of lung cancer? I think to myself. *But he's only 29! How can you go from being told you're healthy to being told you're in the final stages of lung cancer?*

"The day I found out, I didn't speak to my parents about it," he continues. "I had enough strength to tolerate the pain both emotionally and physically because of all the blessings I'd received. I didn't even cry. Now, in the company of my parents I am a little sentimental, but otherwise …"

He pauses.

"I am completely determined to leave this body."

I stare at him, amazed by his bravery.

"I went for radiation. It had so many side effects. They wanted me to do chemotherapy, but I said I didn't want it. I just wanted to do *kirtan* at the Bhubaneswar temple. I'm just ready to leave. I'm going to Bhubaneswar tomorrow, and then, that's it. I have to carry oxygen; without it, I can't fly. Once it is all arranged, I will go. My final journey to Bhubaneswar. I want to see Lord Jagannath, who is so exquisitely and elaborately decorated every night at the Bhubaneswar temple. I am expecting I can go so I can see him. It is my last trip, and then I want to leave my body. Gaur Govinda Swami used to always say, 'If you want to get Krishna, go and cry. Go and cry. He will help you.' I want to go.

"I am strong, but now I need a lot of prayers. You know, I was already engaged to be married? But now, everything has changed. Her name is Badarika. She is so strong, and such an inspiration. She told me, 'Don't think about me, or your parents, or your relatives. Just focus on Jagannath. That's it. Just focus. And get out of this material world. This world is no place for a gentleman.' This is my inspiration. She is in Bhubaneswar right now, waiting for me. She is decorating the rooms with pictures, preparing for my coming back so that my whole attention will be on Krishna. She left her job immediately when she heard I had cancer. I'm very proud that I got such a lady.

"I have been in Bhaktivedanta Hospital for one month. A few days after I arrived, I asked my parents to come here from Orissa.

"Bhaktivedanta Hospital has taken good care of me. They've been managing my pain well so that I can concentrate on Krishna. All the nurses and doctors are very, very nice, and I am so grateful for the way they treat me. And they chant with me. I like it very much. This is the best hospital I've ever seen. They've taken care of me physically, spiritually, and mentally. They offer the complete package so that a patient won't be scared when death comes. It's very nice care. I'm very happy here."

He's very happy here.

"I feel that Srila Prabhupada is more present here than anywhere else in the world, even his temples," I say.

"I agree. And his disciple, Radhanath Swami, has inspired and created this environment," he responds. "People can come here and feel peaceful. People learn so much here, and become free from distress. Otherwise, it is so painful. If someone was told they will die in a couple of months, they'd freak out. 'No, I have to do this, and do that!' No. You just have to remember God. Everything else will be done automatically. So I thank Radhanath Swami and Srila Prabhupada."

For a moment, I don't know what to say or do.

"Is there anything I can do for you?" I say, eventually.

"Are you a writer by profession?" asks Madhava.

"I've been a writer my whole life, but I don't write for a living. This is a volunteer project," I explain. "Would it be okay with you if I include your story in the book?"

"Yes, you can write about me. I'll be happy. That's what you can do for me. You should tell the world about this hospital so that they will also come and see. They will come here, and be treated as whole persons and with love. Here, they are so loving and affectionate."

"Yes, I agree," I say with a smile. "Is there anything else I can do for you?"

"For me? Just pray. Prabhupada said you have to prepare for death. We have to learn the art of dying."

"The faith that you have is exemplary," I say.

"If I can help others, I am happy," he says. "Otherwise, how could I leave this world?"

"What would you like people to know about you?" I ask. "How would you like to be remembered?"

"Don't remember me," Madhava says. "Better to remember Prabhupada, and his teachers before him. Always remember them, and read their books. Don't spend your life trying to make material arrangements to be peaceful, or cozy. This is not the way. We have to read their books. All of them. And through these, you can know Krishna."

After a few moments of silence, I say, "I'd like to give you something." I have the overwhelming urge to give him some sort of gift, but all I have with me is my purse and keys. But I have an idea.

"Lord Jagannath is very dear to me as well. Four years ago on my birthday, a devotee gave me a small gift that I'd like to give to you today. It's really special, and I've been carrying it in my bag since the day I received it."

I reach into my bag, and pull out a button with the face of Lord Jagannath. "He's my good luck charm. And now he's yours."

Madhava's eyes open wide, and his smile widens, "Ahhh," he says. "It's … it's really okay? Thank you so much!"

His eyes light up as he accepts the tiny gift with such gratitude, grace, and joy. It is as though I have given him the world's greatest treasure. I realize, for him, this little button is exactly that.

"Please, I'd like to do something for you—is there anything you need?" I ask.

"You've already given me your good luck charm! Just keep trying to serve Prabhupada and the Bhaktivedanta Hospital," he says. "We need more and more Bhaktivedanta Hospitals, all around the world!"

He pauses for a moment, catching his breath. "Death is a very precious moment," he says after a couple of minutes. "Everyone loses their consciousness. One is shaky at that time. We need strength. Death is the examination time. Real exam. We have to live properly, to die properly. Otherwise, everything is a waste—what is the use? So it will be very helpful if you keep on doing this service. I expect this from you. I feel so nice that a devotee is coming and speaking to me about Krishna, about what they want to do to serve. I wish I could also help you, and I wish I could serve Srila Prabhupada more."

"You have, you are, and you will continue. Beyond this life. Because that is your mood. You are a wonderful devotee," I respond.

I turn to address Madhava's parents.

"Hare Krishna *Mataji* and *Prabhu*. What are your names?" I ask in Hindi.

"Udai," says Madhava's father, who has been quietly listening, smiling, and wiping away tears throughout my conversation with his son.

"My name is Sahaja," says Madhava's mother.

"I'm very honoured to meet you and your son."

For the next few minutes, it's almost as though we temporarily forget the gravity of the situation, and the mood becomes light. Playful, even. Udai shows me his smartphone, of which he is very proud. He tells me about his business ventures and travels. He and Sahaja encourage me when I struggle with finding the right Hindi word. I tell Madhava's parents about my young nephews, and their charming, naughty personalities. They ask questions about life in Canada. We all laugh, and the four of us even take a few pictures together.

Madhava is laughing. He is beautiful. Radiant, even. Then, he becomes pensive.

"There's something else I want to say," he says. "I didn't really have enough time to serve my guru and Krishna. I served from 2007 to 2013, but in between, I lost time. I was an accountant. I worked hard. And now I feel remorse that I didn't do enough, I didn't have enough time. One of my services was to be a driver for my guru and for visiting devotees from out of town. But I wanted more. Now, there are so many projects coming up in Bhubaneswar, and I really wanted to be a part of them. But now, I have not enough time. I always pray to Jagannath—what is your plan? I have millions of plans. But what is *your* plan?

"My guru always says that we should try to understand Krishna's plan and try to fulfill it. I know this is all Krishna's plan. So, I'm happy. I have nothing to worry about. My parents are now more into spiritual life, and all the devotees in Bhubaneswar are fired up to welcome me home. They have arranged everything for me, a complete full package for how to leave the body. That's why I'm very happy. Because they are preparing me to leave. The time of death is the biggest test. This is the only thing I want to say."

"I know Srila Prabhupada is looking after you and wants you to serve him somewhere else. Somewhere different." I say.

"Yes, just not in this body," he responds, with his winning smile.

Udai begins showing me pictures of the rest of the family. Madhava's older sister, married with a son, will be in Bhubaneswar for the passing of her brother.

Sahaja begins to gush about her grandson, and asks me questions about my nephews. "I prayed to Durga Devi[12] for a son, she says. "And," she says, choking up. "She gave me such a beautiful boy."

Sahaja starts to cry. Instinctively, I sit beside her, and hold her hand. I lower my head to kiss her hand, and she unexpectedly pats my head with her right hand, over and

---

12. Durga is a Hindu goddess.

over. It's as if, with this loving gesture, she is blessing me to live a long and happy life, desperately hoping my parents will never have to go through what she is experiencing.

I can't take my hands off her left hand, which I am now holding close to my heart.

Udai asks me to send him the pictures we just took, but there is a technical glitch, and I can't seem to send them. Madhava snatches my phone out of my hands, and tries to show me how to Bluetooth the pictures to his father's phone.

This moment is so beautifully, extraordinarily, ordinary.

"You're just a little bit older than me, like my big sister, my *didi*,"[13] Madhava says playfully.

As if right on cue, I put my hand on his. I know I shouldn't, but at this moment, I do not care.

"Yes, you are my little brother," I say with all the love in my heart.

He puts his hand on my hand, and smiles. "I'm so happy to meet you."

Suddenly, he coughs. A long, deep, horrible, non-stop cough. It's draining him completely as he tries to simply catch his breath and cough at the same time. This continues for minutes. Sahaja rubs his back.

When he is finally able to catch his breath, I say, "I'm so honoured to meet you, Madhava *Prabhu*. I'll leave you with your family now. Thank you so much for speaking with me." An hour has passed.

I want to *say* something, *do* something, but I don't know what.

"All my prayers are with you. I wish you a happy journey close to Srila Prabhupada, and to Lord Jagannath's loving embrace," I muster.

---

13. *Didi* is an affectionate and respectful way to address an older sister.

"Once I go to Orissa, I will run to him, no doubt," he says.

"It's hard for me to leave," I say, feeling grave.

"I understand. Keep serving Prabhupada. Keep writing. Time is limited. *This is your time.* People think money is sweeter than honey," he says, laughing. "It's so useless. Completely useless. Please, *didi*, give me your blessings. I feel very honoured that you've come to speak to me."

"I'm the one who is honoured. Have a safe trip tomorrow. I'll never forget you."

"Don't think of me, think of Krishna," he says, smiling widely again.

I hug Sahaja, and she begins to cry. I hold her, tight. "Please call me if I can do anything for you, okay? I'm keeping you in my prayers," I say softly. I offer my respects to Udai, and leave the room, leaving a piece of my heart behind.

Epilogue

It is now November 2021 as I write this epilogue. It's been almost eight years since I first began this project. I never imagined compiling this book would be as difficult as it was. How do people write multiple books?! I have a newly found respect for every author. I thought this would be simple—transcribe, edit, seek permissions, print. But it was far more complicated than I thought. *Way more.* [Case in point—this book is actually being published a few years after writing this epilogue!]

As I write this, we are in year two of a global pandemic. Bhaktivedanta Hospital has added approximately 100 beds since this project began, and is now officially also a Research Institute. In 2019, they won the PEXA award, which recognizes excellence in patient care. They have expanded their team, and continue to thrive.

As for me, in my travels to India, I spent time with a man who I would ultimately marry. A New Yorker from a Jewish family, who also practices *bhakti*, and we currently live together in the Big City. (There is a whole *Eat, Pray, Love* backstory that is not printed in these pages.)

I didn't imagine a move from Toronto to New York would be difficult—it's Canada and the States, after all. And in many ways, it wasn't. I was able to quickly find a job I love, a *bhakti* community that embraced me, and a family who has always treated me like their own. But, I moved at a time of great political and social unrest, and navigating everyday life in America, and in the Big City, has been challenging, to say the least.

Between gun control, infrastructure, taxes, education, national security, and healthcare, I've suddenly started to care a lot more about politics. These things affect my daily life, more than they ever did whilst living at home, in Toronto. One of the most shocking moments after moving to the States was receiving a bill after visiting a doctor. I was trying to find a Primary Care Physician and went to meet a doctor in a "network" that my insurance accepted (I also didn't know "in" vs. "out" of network was a thing). A few weeks after our meet-and-greet, I received a $100 invoice and was very confused.

Selecting the right insurance plan felt more complicated than rewriting the rules of physics.

I got a bit more up close and personal to the system this year, when, for the first time since beginning this project almost eight years ago, I became a patient.

I should say, my life is not and has not been in any grave danger as a result of this situation.

This Epilogue describes my most recent health episode, an experience that had me longing for the quality of care available at the Bhaktivedanta Hospital, and renewing my resolve that the world would benefit from them expanding their reach.

It all began last summer, with a twitch of my left eye. A little eye twitch never concerned me before. But this didn't really feel normal. I did some research, spoke to my doctor, and we thought the same thing—try to reduce my time in front of the computer, get more sleep. Two things I struggle with regularly, so I didn't think too much of it. It started to get embarrassing, though. We moved to a virtual world, and every time I gave a talk, or participated in a work call, at least one person would say, "Hey what's going on with your eye?" It became quite consistent.

Then, I started to feel like someone was tugging the entire left side of my face. My mouth and even my nose would twitch, consistently. I knew something was wrong. Google suggested Bells Palsy or a hemifacial spasm. I had no clue what was happening to me.

I have grown up in the tradition of *bhakti*, which is rooted in the basic tenet that we are not our bodies. We are spirit souls, separate from the body, which is just a covering of the pure, beautiful, soul.

And yet, this face twitch gave me something of an identity crisis.

I was a little surprised at my own vanity—I've never been someone who cared that much about my physical appearance. It's always been important to me, but until recently I would never have thought of my appearance as something so integral to my sense of self.

But there I was, feeling confused and even betrayed by my body. Questioning my value as a person, as a woman. I had gained a small amount of weight, and was experiencing another minor health issue, and altogether I just started feeling like my body was turning on me.

I know very well that it is a superpower to observe the mind, rather than to identify with it. So, by some wonderful grace, I was able to observe my negative thought patterns—the thought patterns that showed me the slippery slope between body loathing and self-loathing. I wanted to nip these thoughts in the bud before they turned to destructive words or behaviors, so I hired a coach who focuses on body image.

In our first session, my coach told me that many women in their 30s experience slight weight gain; it is the body's way of protecting the bones, which become weaker. This was one small tidbit of information that instantly made me feel better—my body was giving me love, not turning on me.

I went to the doctor for the face twitching, which admittedly was driven more by my vanity than by a concern for my health. Everything I read online indicated that there was no serious health risk. The doctor recommended a neurologist and did a blood test. Before I had the chance to call a neurologist, I received a note from the doctor: "Your calcium is high, which may be a cause for the face twitching. Please visit the lab for some additional blood work."

Who knew excess calcium could lead to something like a face twitch? I read up more on hypercalcemia, and felt a sense of relief to have caught it early. Typical symptoms of high calcium include excessive thirst or confusion—two things I would never have thought to see a doctor for. Suddenly I felt a sense of gratitude for the twitching.

The second blood test was to measure PTH, parathyroid hormone. We each have four parathyroids in the body, typically located just above the thyroid. The job of the parathyroid is to regulate the amount of calcium in the body. When calcium levels are high, doctors check for one or more overactive parathyroid gland by measuring PTH. As expected, my PTH levels were high.

Next, I was sent to an endocrinologist, Dr. W, who was wonderful. She predicted that mine was a classic case of a benign tumour in one or more of the parathyroids, causing hyperactivity, causing the high calcium and the face twitching. She would send me for imaging exams, and told me that the remedy would be surgery. She said it was a simple day surgery, with a quick recovery, and that it was very common. There would be a scar on my neck, relatively small, and that with some careful nursing could be unrecognizable after about a year. She made me feel very calm, and unafraid. I was relieved to be getting to the bottom of what was happening to my body. She told me that while surgery wouldn't be urgent, better to take care of it sooner rather than later, because excess calcium could later lead to other problems, including with the kidneys.

Cool. I was ready to get rid of this embarrassing twitch as

soon as possible. To not have to apologize for keeping my camera off on client calls, or to not have people stare when the twitch would start.

I got an ultrasound and CT Scan of the neck. Both indicated some enlargement of at least one parathyroid, and a miniscule tumour. I went to see the surgeon, Dr. K. He was lovely. He was dressed in a professional suit, was very kind, calm, methodical. He did some additional imaging and was very gentle. Whereas in the lab I found the technicians to be a bit sloppy with the ultrasound gel, and rather impersonal, Dr. K was gentle, clean, and very calming. He confirmed that he was seeing something on the top right parathyroid and that we should remove it. He told me that he would remove one parathyroid; then while I'm still on the operating table, he would measure the calcium levels. If they wouldn't decrease to the acceptable amount, he would explore more and potentially remove another, and repeat until calcium levels would be acceptable. We can each survive with half of one parathyroid, he said.

He added that after surgery, it would take a few weeks for everything to stabilize. He said that high calcium could tend to make people feel depressed. I am grateful to not be prone to depression. But wow—what effects could this have on my personality?

I went home that day and told my husband that if I could, I would make Dr. K my doctor for everything. He spent a lot of time with me, didn't make me feel rushed, answered all my questions. It was early October, and he said I could expect surgery to be in early November, and that we'd schedule it right away, otherwise his calendar gets booked quickly. On the way out, Dr. K's assistant walked me to the reception area, and told the staff there that I'd need to schedule one pre-operative test for clearance, and also that we should try to schedule surgery sooner rather than later. The receptionist acknowledged me, and said that there was nothing more for me to do—she would arrange that pre-operative test and then contact me to schedule surgery.

About a week passed, and I didn't hear anything. I called the office and left a message. I didn't hear back. I sent an email to Dr. K's assistant, and asked if maybe I had misunderstood; was I supposed to call someone to schedule that pre-operative exam? Or was I waiting to hear back? The assistant wrote back saying she would follow up with reception—it was their job to contact me to schedule the test. I thanked her.

Another week passed. I was confused. I had updated my family and friends that I would need surgery, and everyone was asking me when it would be. I also needed to make arrangements to take time off work. I left another message, with a person. No response. Finally, I reached the woman in charge of scheduling. "Oh sure, yeah, I am putting the request through. Oh, you want to schedule the surgery now, too? Okay. It will be either on the 1st or the 3rd. You don't have to call me back, okay? I'll call you to confirm the date. Okay? Bye." I was rushed off the phone. It dawned on me that had I not followed up with her, she would not have proactively scheduled the surgery. I had been in anxiety, with a sense of uncertainty, and there was no acknowledgment that she had made a mistake.

I got the clearance from the pre-operative test, and then had to chase the scheduler to confirm the date of the surgery—again. Was it on the 1st? The 3rd? I managed to reach the scheduler, and was met with the same indifference and urgency to get off the phone. "Yeah, you're scheduled on the 3rd, we already talked about that."

No, we didn't. You were supposed to call me to confirm the date. I thought to myself.

After knowing the date of surgery, I felt a little better. Now that I had a date, I could plan for it. My husband, a busy co-founder, could plan for it. My parents-in-law could plan for it. My friends who wanted to help could plan for it. There were so many moving pieces, and all I needed was a date. In the end, it was confirmed a week ahead of time.

I knew in my heart that this was a relatively minor surgery. But it was still a little scary that they were going to cut my neck open. I told my husband everything I wanted should I leave my body. I didn't think anything would go wrong, but I still thought to tell him, almost in passing, what to do with my personal affairs should anything go wrong. "My editor has the latest copy of *Magic on Mira Road*; please work with him to publish it," was one of my main instructions.

The day before surgery, I got the call that I should arrive at 6 a.m., and that surgery would be at 7:30 a.m. My husband could come with me in the morning, which I was grateful for, given our new COVID world.

It is now the day of surgery.

I wake up just before 5 a.m. I look at my neck in a mirror. Such a feminine part of the body. *It will never be the same after today*, I think to myself. A beat later, I have a shower, and offer my prayers. It is the holy month of *Kartik*, so I offer a lamp to Krishna and his mother, as this month honours Krishna's childhood pastimes. I water my *tulasi* plant, say a number of prayers, and head out in a cab, together with Hari, my husband. I am more grateful than ever that he is by my side. We hold hands and chant *japa* on the way to the hospital.

We arrive a few minutes early, and check in with a friendly receptionist who asks me to sign some forms about my insurance. We sit in the waiting room, where after a few moments a lovely nurse called Andrea collects me. She asks

Hari to wait for a few moments and tells him she will call him shortly.

Andrea leads me through a door and down a corridor, into a room with a number of patients all sectioned by curtains. We arrive in the last "room" and I am asked to sit in a comfortable chair while she takes a seat in front of her computer. She asks me some standard questions ("Tell me in your own words what you're having done today."), and then asks me to brush my teeth, change into a hospital gown, and wear a hairnet. She takes my vitals and calls Hari to the room. I am feeling vulnerable, wearing a hospital gown and socks, a mask, and a hairnet.

I can hear the conversation happening with the patient beside us—after all, we are only sectioned off by a thin curtain. He is having some sort of arm surgery, I gather. He is alone. He could hear everything we are saying, and we can likewise hear everything he is saying. I keep thinking about Bhaktivedanta Hospital. What I wouldn't give for some spiritual care right now. I chant the Nrismhadeva Prayers, prayers for protection.

Then, a man with a loud voice abruptly, and loudly, opens the curtain to our "room," and says, "Hi, I'm Dr. Y, your anesthesiologist." He barely looks at me. He is clearly in a rush. Rapid fire, he asks me all the questions he needs to ask. He is not looking at me—he is marking my answers on the computer. I try to make a little small talk. "Do I detect an Australian accent?" I ask. We chit-chat a little about where we're from. Not a minute later, he pulls out an iPad, and asks me to sign. He has clicked the "sign" button and says, "This form just says we talked about the anesthesia you're having."

"Do you mind if I have a quick read before I sign?" I ask.

"Sure, of course," he says, as he unclicks the "sign" button, which allows me to read. I can tell he doesn't have time for me to read. He is fidgety. I have a quick skim of the document, and I sign, returning it to Dr. Y for his signature. He signs, and then the iPad dies.

"Oh my God! This happens all the time!" he says in a loud voice. "Ugh, I apologize. F***! This always happens and it's such a waste of time! I apologize, I'll be right back."

He leaves the room, opening the curtains and not closing them. We hear him on the other side of the room complaining about the iPad. My husband is amused. I am not. Dr. Y is not unfriendly; but his energy makes me uncomfortable.

Dr. Y returns (and of course, without "knocking"), asks me to re-sign, and says, without looking at me, "Sorry about that, see you in there!" And just like that, he grabs the iPad and disappears. He does not close the curtains behind him. Andrea reappears, and says, "Dr. K is on his way to see you now, okay?"

"Okay, thank you," Hari and I say. We are both chanting *japa*.

A few moments later, Dr. K knocks, shakes Hari's hand, and sits at the chair. I'm happy to see him.

"You ready?" he says with a smile.

"I guess so," I say, returning his smile.

His face crinkles. "Well, we spent a lot of time preparing, didn't we?" His answer strikes me as a little odd; yes, we did—but I can still be nervous, can't I?

"Yes," I say, smiling awkwardly behind my mask.

"So here's what will happen," he says. "Based on the imaging, we think we need to remove the parathyroid on the upper right. As soon as we remove it, we will measure your calcium levels, while you're still on the table. We will take a little blood, send it to the lab, and they will return the results right away. Hopefully, the calcium drops to the appropriate level, and we're done. That is Plan A. If the calcium levels do not drop as much as we'd like, we'll check to see if any other parathyroid needs to be removed. The imaging indicated there might be an enlarged parathyroid on the bottom left as well. Removing a second parathyroid is Plan B. If your calcium levels still don't drop, we can do Plan C and remove a third parathyroid, but we really don't think we'll need to do that."

I ask about where exactly the incision will be. He answers, and then tells Hari he'll call him once the surgery is over.

"Okay, I'll see you in there!" he says. He pats Hari's shoulder and leaves.

We continue our *japa*.

A few moments later, Andrea reappears. "Okay, you ready? Let's go," she says. She takes my bag of belongings and says she will have them ready for me in Recovery. Hari walks with us outside of the room, across a corridor, and then up to a set of large double doors.

"Okay, Hari, this is where we'll ask you to exit, and she will see you after the surgery."

Hari and I look at each other. This is the first time my eyes water. He smiles, and he hugs me tightly. "Love you so much," he says. "Everything will be perfect. I'll see you this afternoon." I bury my face into his neck, wrap my arms around him, and then let go. I give him a little smile and wave, and then walk through the large doors with Andrea.

I notice I am holding my hands in front of me and clenching my fists. Andrea can tell I am nervous, so she attempts to calm me by placing her left arm around me and her right hand on my arm as we walk. I am more grateful than I can say at that moment; I genuinely feel comforted by her.

We arrive to O. R. 7. Andrea knocks on the door.

"Hi!" An extremely bubbly, beautiful woman answers

the door. "Welcome to your humble abode for the next few hours! I'm Natalie," she says. Andrea says goodbye, and I walk inside with Natalie. I smile at her. "Hi," I say.

"Don't mind the hip hop in the background," Natalie says, as she points to a stereo. "Dr. K LOVES his hip hop! He like, gets angry if we don't have hip hop on in the room!" she says with a laugh.

In the days before surgery I thought about asking if we could play some *kirtan* in the O. R., but I didn't want to impose. But this, I really didn't expect.

"Come on over, and have a seat on the table," Natalie says.

There is another man in the room who is doing something on a table. He turns and smiles at me. Dr. Y is behind the bed, fiddling with something. He is with another woman, who seems to be a student, and they both say hello. Natalie loosens my gown slightly from the back and asks me to lie down on the table. She gently places a blanket over me, and then puts a tube under the blanket that blows out hot air to keep me warm. There is chit-chat, laughter, and hip hop in the background. I feel like I'm entering a party. It's almost 7:30 a.m. On a Wednesday.

The woman who is working with the anesthesiologist says, "So I hear you're from Toronto? I am too!" We small talk a little about the neighbourhoods we grew up in. In my mind, I'm still a little thrown off by the hip hop. I actually like hip hop (though I always preferred RnB), but this is weird.

Dr. Y has to lower the top of the bed and he does it with a jerk. He doesn't say anything to me. He asks me to stretch out my arm, and he starts flicking my hand to get a vein. He is not gentle. Natalie is trying to distract me with small talk. She is very bubbly. Dr. Y is teaching the other woman how to insert an IV. It hurts.

"Ugh, her vein is so small; we're going to have to try the

other side. Sorry."

"Oh, no problem," I say, though I'm quite sure he wasn't talking to me.

Dr. Y is saying something about this not being his day, or him being frustrated, or something along those lines. They come to the other side, and flick my hand again, and not gently. "Sorry," says Dr. Y, "this will bruise."

"It's okay," I say.

"Shall we just give her the baseline?" Natalie says.

What's a baseline? I think to myself.

Dr. K enters the room. It's about 7:32 a.m.

"Sorry," says Natalie to Dr. K. "Almost ready. We couldn't get a good vein."

"Sure," says Dr. K. He does not acknowledge me.

Dr. Y drops something on my left, and grunts loudly. Dr. K picks it up and gives it to him.

"You're going to start feeling a little out of it now," says Dr. Y.

I start to pray. I'm starting to feel a little like the room is spinning. I pray first to Srimati Radharani, the divine feminine, and then to Lord Nrismhadeva, for protection.

And that's that.

༚ ༚ ༚ ༚

"Can you tell me on a scale of 1-10 your pain level?" I hear.

I am insanely groggy. Am I awake? I give a number, maybe 6. I think I hear someone say, "Okay, we want you to be at a 4 or below so we will give you some medication."

I'm not sure if I dreamed that. I am so out of it. Just in and out of sleep.

The next thing I know, I am in Recovery. I have no recollection of how I got there.

There is a nurse; he tells me his name is Jason. With all my Canadianisms, all I remember saying is, "Please," and "Thank you," a lot.

The first time I am a little conscious, I ask for a mirror. I want to see the incision. Jason hands me my phone, and I turn on the camera, and point it at myself.

Holy cow. It is huge. Much bigger than I thought it would be. Darker. My face is still twitching. My face is still twitching. I could cry, but I can't keep my eyes open.

I pass out again.

At one point I ask for water. My throat is so dry. I feel like I've never had water in my life.

I ask for some lip balm. My lips are chapped.

I had been intubated for surgery, making my voice soft and hoarse, and my throat and lips dry.

At one point, Jason asks me to eat some apple sauce so I can take some medication. Somehow, I am able to eat a couple of bites. Then I pass out. After that, a couple more bites. Then take the medicine Jason is giving me. Have some water. Pass out again. Is that a blood pressure monitor on my arm? Yes, it must be. They must be measuring my vitals. I cannot keep my eyes open.

I think Dr. K comes in. I say, "Thank you" to him in my sleep. I think he's trying to talk to me, but I can't stay awake.

Jason asks me if I can please move onto a chair. I do as I'm told. I think I'm sleepwalking. Jason helps me onto a chair.

I pass out.

I wake up at one point to say, "Does this recline? Can you recline this a little?"

Then I pass out again.

It seems the curtains are open and everyone who is walking by can see me. *Why can't they just close the darn curtain?* I think to myself. But I'm not conscious enough to ask for it.

I open my eyes again, and Hari is here. "Hari, I love you," I say.

"I love you!" he says back with a smile. I'm so happy to see him.

"My face is still twitching," I say.

"I know, honey," he says.

And then I'm asleep again.

And so the pattern continues. Jason walks me through some of the medications I'm supposed to be on, but honestly, I have no idea what he's talking about.

Finally, I'm a little more conscious. I ask Jason, "Hey, what did Dr. K do? How many parathyroids did he remove?"

"One," says Hari. "He called me and said everything went well, and that he stuck to Plan A."

"Actually," says Jason as he looks at his computer, "it looks like they removed two parathyroids on the right."

"Oh really? Did I misunderstand?" asks Hari.

I am confused, but don't have the wherewithal to ask questions.

Jason is saying it's time to go home. He removes the blood pressure monitor. "I'm going to remove five stickers from your body now, okay?" And he proceeds to remove five stickers near my chest.

Hari walks me to the washroom where I change into my own clothes. I notice a little bulge in my sock. What is that? I remove the sock, and peel off another sticker and a large cotton ball.

Jason tells us to go to the pharmacy in the hospital to pick up painkillers and calcium supplements.

Wait, why do I need calcium supplements? I think to myself.

But I'm too out of it to ask. Jason asks if I'll need a wheelchair to leave. "No thank you," I say. But I'm so dizzy, and so groggy, so he insists, and I relent.

Another gentleman arrives with a wheelchair. He does not acknowledge me. Jason puts a document in my bag, my "After Visit Summary." I thank him for all his help. But before I finish my sentence, the gentleman swings my chair the other way, towards the elevators, and I need to close my eyes because the movement is making me dizzier.

I was in surgery until almost 10 a.m. I was in Recovery for just over three hours.

I am dizzy in the elevator. I am dizzy and tired in the pharmacy. I am dizzy and asleep in the cab. We come home, and I sleep for a couple of hours.

My parents-in-law arrive with dinner. I feel much better. I don't need to hold a hand while I walk anymore; the dizziness has largely gone away, and I feel like I could get up, walk around, and talk. My throat is in pain. I'm a little slow to move, but I'm okay. I know that my throat is sore because I was intubated, and that tomorrow and the next day, I'll feel much better. A couple of friends come visit in the evening with their two-year old daughter (I insist it's okay), and they also drop off some food.

By the time everyone leaves, it is about 10:30 p.m. I have slept all day. I'm tired, but I'm not sleepy. Hari cleans up, we both offer our evening lamp and chant some more *japa*. Hari says he will go to bed and asks if I'm coming. "I think I need to write," I tell him. He kisses me goodnight, and I grab my journal and a pen. I write down all of what happened in the day.

All seems to have gone well with surgery. But I feel something churning inside me—I'm feeling uneasy and I'm trying to articulate why.

According to Jason, Dr. K removed two parathyroids on the right. The imaging suggested one enlarged on the right, and potentially one on the left. So what exactly happened? Isn't that something they should have told me before I left? It feels funny that they cut my neck open and now that I'm home, I don't know what they took out.

And I know it's a small thing, but—why was there a sticker on my foot? Surgery was on my neck, so what were they doing at my foot? While I was unconscious, someone removed my sock, put something on my foot, and then put my sock back on. I know it's not a big deal, but I just didn't expect that.

Did they have to remove the top of my gown to put the stickers near my chest? Who did that? Was I exposed? And while there was hip hop on in the room?

I thought it would be about a 2cm incision, but this is definitely bigger. Maybe I misunderstood. And it's much higher than I thought; I won't be able to hide this with my neck beads. And—the twitch hasn't gone away. Does this mean it is not due to high calcium? Or does it just need to stabilize? Will it ever go away? Why do I need more calcium; I thought the point of the surgery was to reduce it? These calcium supplements are making me feel a little head-achey and queasy. And maybe even a little loopy. Or maybe that's the anesthesia. Regardless, I don't feel like myself.

Will my body react okay to this procedure? Is this scar going to heal nicely?

I know this surgery was necessary to prevent future problems. But, did I need to do it now? I was driven in large part by my vanity to have this surgery, and now I have a large incision on my neck and the twitching is still happening. Did I just opt to feel even more insecure about my appearance?

One thing that's making me feel better, is that I'm genuinely feeling carried by people's prayers. Even if I'm not special, I know the people who are praying for me are.

I guess I'm still kind of processing the emotions. I haven't really had the chance to. I think Hari is a little overwhelmed with all he had to do today—between answering all the calls and texts he received about me, finding a vegetarian calcium supplement, dealing with random bizarre things that happened in our flat today (a blown fuse! With a spark!), trying to fend off work, feeling worried about me. I feel a little guilty. A little like a burden. I know Hari does not at all feel burdened, nor does he want me to feel any guilt.

I feel very loved.

I feel confused.

I feel grateful.

I feel sad.

I feel worried that maybe I did something wrong.

I feel scared about the total lack of control over my health.

I feel worried about the scar.

I feel a little uneasy towards Dr. K and Dr. Y. How is Dr. K going to enjoy hip hop while opening up my neck? Does he really get angry if there's no hip hop in the room? Something about that—it feels like a wrestler entering his ring, with his preferred music to hype him up. It's about winning. It's about conquering.

Somehow I feel slightly violated.

I feel so deeply vulnerable because I don't know what they did while I was unconscious on their table.

I feel exploited.

I feel tired.

I feel drained.

I feel carried by the love and prayers of others. I don't know how—it's noetic.

Dear Krishna, I'm so sorry to ask—but at this actual instant the twitching prevents me from seeing properly so please may I ask you to remove it? I know people suffer so much more than this and I don't want to be entitled—but for me, this is hard.

I look to the 15-page "After Visit Summary" again to see if it has more answers to my questions. It tells me to expect some pain, to not remove the dressing from the wound. It tells me I can resume normal physical activity as soon as I'm up for it. I should schedule my follow-up appointment as soon as possible. It gives me some tips on controlling pain. The rest of the document is about the painkillers and the calcium supplements. What are the side effects, when to call a doctor. Oh, it turns out I should expect to feel head-achey and even a little confused. Next, it tells me who to call if I have questions about my bills.

And then, two more phone numbers—the National Suicide Prevention Hotline and the NYC Suicide Hotline. These numbers are listed under "Additional Resources."

Are you kidding me? Is this the only recognition that there is an emotional component to healing?

A nurse calls me the next day to see how I'm feeling. I have a few questions about how and when to nurse the scar. I'm still a little confused and groggy. I ask her what the doctor removed—it's my most pressing question.

"You can ask that in your follow-up appointment, or you can try emailing Dr. K," she says.

Okay.

And with that, she says, "Hope you feel better soon!" and hangs up. I wasn't quite done.

I email Dr. K to ask him about my scar, and about what he removed.

It is now 9 days after surgery. I emailed Dr. K six days ago, and have not heard back.

The doctors did a wonderful job of taking care of me physically; there is no doubt. Maybe some of you read that experience and felt that it was perfectly lovely. And it was. They did their job, and they were kind.

But, I can't stop thinking about how helpful it would have been if I could have stayed a little longer at the hospital, and had access to the information I was seeking. I felt a little rushed out—like they needed the bed—the chair—they had me on. A little Canadian voice in me is wondering if this surgery was necessary at all—did they just do this for money? It didn't even stop the twitching. Did I make a mistake?

And I keep remembering the patients at Bhaktivedanta Hospital who told me how soothing it was to have devotional music playing prior to a procedure. To have that same music playing during and afterwards. To have doctors who clearly have a service mentality, who genuinely see themselves as instruments of the Divine—not as conquerors, or controllers, or wrestlers in an arena. How powerful it is to be in that atmosphere, that is intentional and rooted in wisdom and prayer.

I understand why Bhaktivedanta Hospital emphasizes that their staff must be aware of how they come across—their facial expressions, the tones of their voices, their mannerisms—and how a seemingly innocent gesture, or word, can affect a patient and her family deeply. And ultimately her healing.

I understand why patients said they felt half healed just by being in the atmosphere of Bhaktivedanta Hospital. Why people really felt that the physical aspect of their health was just that—one aspect. That they are whole people.

How much I long for a healthcare practitioner, someone who understands what I just went through, to talk to me. Just an ear to help me process the emotionality behind such seemingly small things like—having a scar. Not understanding why there was a sticker on my foot and how something so silly and small actually made me feel deeply vulnerable. To understand that it makes me feel powerless that I don't know what they took out of my body.

I needed someone to tell me before surgery that my symptoms wouldn't disappear right away. That there would be five stickers near my chest when I woke up. That I'd be on calcium supplements.

And the more people I share this story with, the more stories I hear, sadly, of patients who didn't feel like they were treated as humans, with the full dignity they longed for.

A man who was convinced by his doctors to have a surgery but then found out after the fact that the long-term consequences for him meant painkillers for life.

A woman whose egg retrieval went wrong, whose doctors didn't tell her about it, and who now lives with excruciating pain and cannot do anything about it because the hospital could sue her for defamation.

A woman who miscarried and felt invisible during dilation and evacuation—the removal of a dead fetus from her womb.

A man with cancer who passed away after being denied coverage by his health insurance carrier.

A woman who lost her father and couldn't get any of the doctors and nurses to clearly answer her questions about how he passed.

There are *too many stories.*

I was reflecting on how minor my procedure was, in the grand scheme of things. I keep thinking about cancer patients who have multiple surgeries. About the feeling of your body not being yours. Of your body just being a specimen. Something fascinating for scientists to explore. Of the sheer emotionality behind the scars.

Now, living in the US, thinking about the bills that we will need to pay—not having a clue what that bill will be, and how much my insurance will cover.

There is *so much to process.*

The absence of emotional and spiritual support genuinely prolongs the healing journey. I can feel it.

It's very important for me to say, that I am deeply grateful for my healthcare providers. I don't believe they did anything wrong (except for not being clear about what they did). I'm confident that my experience was better than those of others. I had an experienced and kind surgeon, and very friendly people in the room, some of whom really tried their best to make me feel comfortable. I had a lovely nurse, and am grateful that they called the next day to check on me. The After Visit Summary was very helpful and explained some of what I was feeling. My "network" is one of the best in the country. And some might argue that it's not the doctors' job to worry about the patients' emotions—and, to an extent, that may be true.

Especially now, in the midst of this global pandemic, it is so important for me to emphasize this—our healthcare workers, to me, are superheroes. I can't imagine being in their shoes, and the emotionality behind their roles. The kinds of things they see. They don't have the kind of support the doctors at Bhaktivedanta Hospital have—dedicated care programs to prevent compassion fatigue. Different measures of performance that encourage holistic care. Globally, most doctors work in systems that set them up to be impersonal. Or motivated by the wrong things. Maybe they want to provide more empathy but their metrics prevent them from being able to do so. In fact, I know this to be true—I have enough friends in the healthcare industry to know that sometimes, they're not allowed to spend as much time as they want to with the patient. Some of them tell me that they too, feel like robots, and not humans, due to the systems in which they work. All they're able to do is address the bodily need; they simply don't have time to handle the emotions. They are measured strictly on competency, and not character.

By contrast, the Spiritual Care team at Bhaktivedanta Hospital is solely dedicated to this—to talk, to listen. To address the patient as a whole person. They truly are the heart of the hospital. The need for authentic, loving care within hospitals, and healthcare in general, is not unique to the United States. It is prevalent in Canada, India, and around the world.

Now, more than ever, I can appreciate the Bhaktivedanta Hospital, and just how important and effective their mission is. To receive holistic care at a time like this, would have been life-changing.[1]

It's time to finally change the conversation. To truly embrace holistic care, worldwide. To critically analyze how healthcare practitioners are rewarded, and how people actually heal.

When I began this project, I had no idea what to expect. I just decided to accept a challenge, and to go on an adventure. I had always wanted to write books, and this was a great story just waiting to be told.

What I found instead, was a sense of purpose. A story that was bigger than me, a cause that was so pure. I was humbled, realizing my great fortune to be the one writing this story, even though it's not my story to tell. I was invited to participate in something greater—a movement, a miracle. *Magic*.

I felt small—not insignificant, but small in the way one feels when gazing up at a beautiful mountain, in awe of its magnificence and mystery.

Soon after returning from the Bhaktivedanta Hospital, I attended a class during a major celebration in the *bhakti* tra-

---

[1]. At the time of the latest edit (2025), my calcium levels have normalized, and I have a diagnosis of a hemifacial spasm. I am working with doctors to understand the cause and to explore different treatment options.

dition. The speaker asked us to draw a picture of the change we wanted to see in the world and how we could contribute.

In the world I dreamed of, doctors from across the globe volunteer their time and expertise at the Bhaktivedanta Hospital. Non-medical volunteers serve at the camps for impoverished communities. Healthcare administrators around the world collaborate with the hospital to implement holistic care in their own medical facilities. The hospital is invited to set up operations at refugee camps. The origin story of the hospital is immortalized in books and films. Countless people are empowered to heal holistically, and be physically, spiritually, emotionally, and socially healthy. Srila Prabhupada is further celebrated for his immense contributions to health, spirituality, culture, education, sustainable living, and fostering unity across religious, social, and cultural lines.

I don't know if any of this will come to fruition. I don't even know if this book will reach anyone beyond the staff at the hospital and my family and friends.

But perhaps this small offering can serve as the seed of something greater—a future where compassion, service, and care know no boundaries. A future where each of us is called to our greater purpose: to serve one another with intention and love, regardless of any bodily designation, in accordance with universal spiritual principles.

If this vision resonates with you, I encourage you to make the effort to take care of your own holistic health, and to help others do the same. I also encourage you to visit bhaktivedantahospital.com and consider offering your time, expertise, or support to help continue the critical work taking place at the Bhaktivedanta Hospital.

Let's make the most of our time by making an impact—by caring for each other, body, mind, and soul. As Madhava said, "Time is limited. *This* is your time."

Acknowledgments

Radhanath Swami—Thank you for being the visionary behind the Bhaktivedanta Hospital. Your kindness, compassion, and desire for a harmonious world permeate the walls of the hospital in such a meaningful, tangible, and yet mystical way. I am deeply grateful to you.

Niranjana Swami—Thank you for having a vision to publish the stories of the staff and patients of Bhaktivedanta Hospital, and for having the trust and faith in me to try and execute your vision. You are the exemplar of care and an inspiration to all.

Candramauli Swami—Thank you for your consistent encouragement and tolerance all these years, and for the infinite blessings you've poured on me to complete this project.

Giriraj Swami—Thank you for your fatherly love and support for this project.

Dr. Ajay Sankhe, Dr. Girish Rathod, Dr. Dhaval Dalal, Dr. Vivek Shanbhag—I will be forever indebted to you for trusting me with this project, and for your incredible hospitality while I stayed at Bhaktivedanta Hospital and all the years since. In your presence I feel like a treasured family member, and I know that's how all the people in your lives, including your patients, feel every day. As Radhanath Swami said, for the enormous service of founding this hospital, you will be remembered for the whole of history.

Shraboni Sen, Vinay Krishna, Vihan Krishna—Thank you for letting me crash at your home almost every weekend for months while I was living in Mumbai. This project would not be complete without your loving hospitality and care.

Vraja and Kasper Waclawski—I only had the opportunity to do this service because you connected me to Niranjana Swami. I will always be indebted to you for changing my life.

Steven Rosen—Thank you not only for your expert editing, but also for pushing me to keep this project afloat.

Anna Cooperberg—Thank you for your edit of the first draft of this manuscript. This book is better because of your exceptional talent.

Mayapriya Long—Thank you for believing in this project and for serving with such sincerity and dedication.

Mom, Dad, Anjali, Gopal, Kumari, Shaan, Jai, Anjaneya Rupa—Thank you for always tolerating my urge to hop on a plane and travel for months at a time, and for fully cheerleading all my adventures. You are the steady foundation of all that I do.

Aba and Ima—Thank you for making me feel like the most talented writer on the planet, even when I clearly am not! Your faith in me makes me feel like I can fly.

Hari—There is no bigger cheerleader, no better support, no better shoulder to cry on than yours (and there were a lot of tears and existential crises in putting together this book!). Thank you for listening to this book, chapter by chapter, and giving me notes that have made this offering the best it possibly can be. You are a gifted writer and editor. Thank you for being my best friend, even in all the behind-the-scenes boule de cristal moments. Je t'aime.

To all my friends who have ever provided a supportive word, who have asked about the progress of this manuscript, who provided feedback on stories—Thank you for keeping me going. In particular, to Nirakula Devi (my oxygen), and to Edward Anobah (my friend, big brother, and mentor)—thank you.

To the patients and patient families who shared their stories with me—thank you, from the bottom of my heart, for sharing so openly and vulnerably with me. Thank you for being brave enough to share your experiences, that will no doubt touch the hearts of all who read this book. I'm beyond grateful that you let me into your lives.

To all the staff at the Bhaktivedanta Hospital, including those whose stories made it into the manuscript, and those whose didn't—thank you for inviting me into your home. Thank you for making yourselves vulnerable, for sharing your inspiration. Thank you for making me feel like family. Thank you for imbibing the love that Radhanath Swami and Srila Prabhupada have for all of humanity, and paying it forward on their behalf. May your service continue to inspire the masses for many years to come.

And finally, Srila Prabhupada—thank you, for being the inspiration behind this hospital. For risking your life to save all of ours. For having a vision that can unite the whole of humanity, regardless of any bodily designation. Thank you for sprinkling your magic on the Bhaktivedanta Hospital every day, and for letting me witness it firsthand for a couple of glorious months.

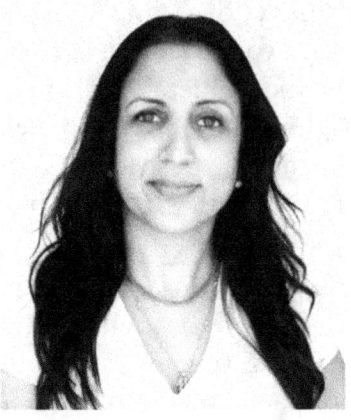

In 2013, Radha Bhakti Dasi travelled to India to learn more about the Bhaktivedanta Hospital and discovered a calling to explore how healthcare and spirituality intersect. She is a writer, management consultant, and speaker living in New York City with her husband. *Magic on Mira Road* is her debut book, inviting readers to reflect on holistic health while learning a little about the wisdom of *bhakti-yoga*—a path that is mystical yet grounded in knowledge, infused with compassion, and open to all. Follow Radha Bhakti on Instagram @radha.bhakti.108.

www.ingramcontent.com/pod-product-compliance
Lightning Source LLC
Chambersburg PA
CBHW071153070526
44584CB00019B/2777